NEW NOTES ON NURSING

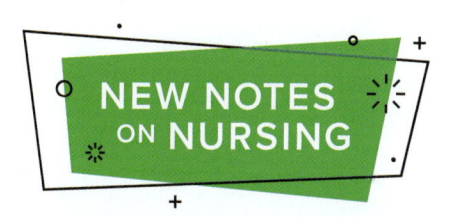

NURSING PROFESSIONALISM FOR NURSING STUDENTS

NEW NOTES ON NURSING

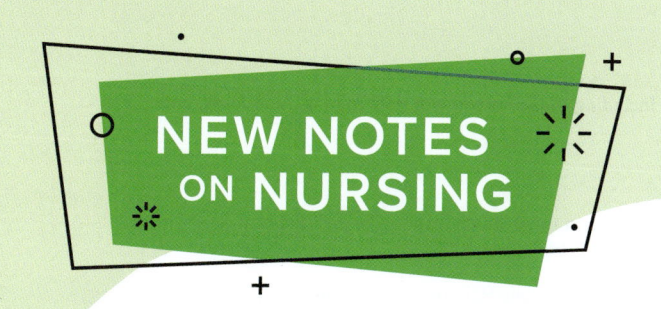

NURSING PROFESSIONALISM FOR NURSING STUDENTS

EDITOR

Tara Iles, RN, BSc (Hons), MSc, MSc

SERIES EDITOR

Teresa Chinn, MBE, RN, QN

CONSULTING EDITOR

June Girvin

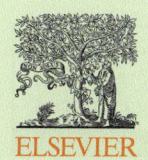

ELSEVIER

© 2026, Elsevier Limited. All rights are reserved, including those for text and data mining, AI training, and similar technologies.

First edition 2026

Publisher's note: *Elsevier* takes a neutral position with respect to territorial disputes or jurisdictional claims in its published content, including in maps and institutional affiliations.

No part of this publication may be reproduced or transmitted in any form or by any means, electronic or mechanical, including photocopying, recording, or any information storage and retrieval system, without permission in writing from the publisher. Details on how to seek permission, further information about the Publisher's permissions policies and our arrangements with organizations such as the Copyright Clearance Center and the Copyright Licensing Agency, can be found at our website: www.elsevier.com/permissions

This book and the individual contributions contained in it are protected under copyright by the Publisher (other than as may be noted herein).

Notices

Practitioners and researchers must always rely on their own experience and knowledge in evaluating and using any information, methods, compounds or experiments described herein. Because of rapid advances in the medical sciences, in particular, independent verification of diagnoses and drug dosages should be made. To the fullest extent of the law, no responsibility is assumed by Elsevier, authors, editors or contributors for any injury and/or damage to persons or property as a matter of products liability, negligence or otherwise, or from any use or operation of any methods, products, instructions, or ideas contained in the material herein.

ISBN: 978-0-323-93140-3

Printed in India
Last digit is the print number: 9 8 7 6 5 4 3 2 1

Content Strategist: Robert Edwards
Content Project Manager: Supriya Barua
Design: Miles Hitchen
Marketing Manager: Deborah J. Watkins

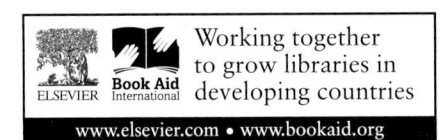

Working together to grow libraries in developing countries
www.elsevier.com • www.bookaid.org

CONTRIBUTORS

Ruth Bailey, MSc, BSc (Hons), RGN, DFSRH, FRT, Onc Cert, QN

Philip Ball, MA, RN, rtd., Dip. Nursing, BSc (Hons)

Robin Binks, MSc, BSc

Nick Browning, MSc, BSc (Hons)

Katharine Caddick, MSc Advanced Practice, BSc (Hons), Nursing NMP, Florence Nightingale Scholar

Sandra Dilks, MSc, RGN, SPPN, PGCE

Heidi Dine, MSc, BSc (Hons), RN, QN

Liz Grogan, MSc, Dip in Adult Nursing

Debra Hazeldine, MBE

Sarah Jarvis, MSc, BSc (Hons)

Hayley Jones, MSc, BSc

Penelope Millington, ENMH and RNMH (now known as RNLD), PGD, PBS, MA

Michelle Samson, MSc, DipHE Nursing Studies, BSc (Hons), PGCert Leadership and Management, PGCert Specialist Practice

TABLE OF CONTENTS

ABOUT THE SERIES, xi

ABOUT THIS BOOK, xvii

1. NOTES ON BEING PROFESSIONAL AND BEING A PROFESSIONAL, 3

2. NOTES ON DEFINING PROFESSIONALISM, 25

3. NOTES ON PROFESSIONALISM AND THE NMC, 53

4. NOTES ON RAISING CONCERNS IDENTIFYING UNPROFESSIONALISM AND MAINTAINING SAFETY, 81

5. NOTES ON BARRIERS AND ENABLERS TO NURSING PROFESSIONALISM, 111

6. NOTES ON PERSONAL VERSUS PROFESSIONAL, 137

7. NOTES ON DIGITAL PROFESSIONALISM, 163

8. NOTES ON WHAT BEING A PROFESSIONAL LOOKS LIKE, 193

9. NOTES ON PROFESSIONAL NURSING: BEYOND THE CODE, 229

MIND MAP

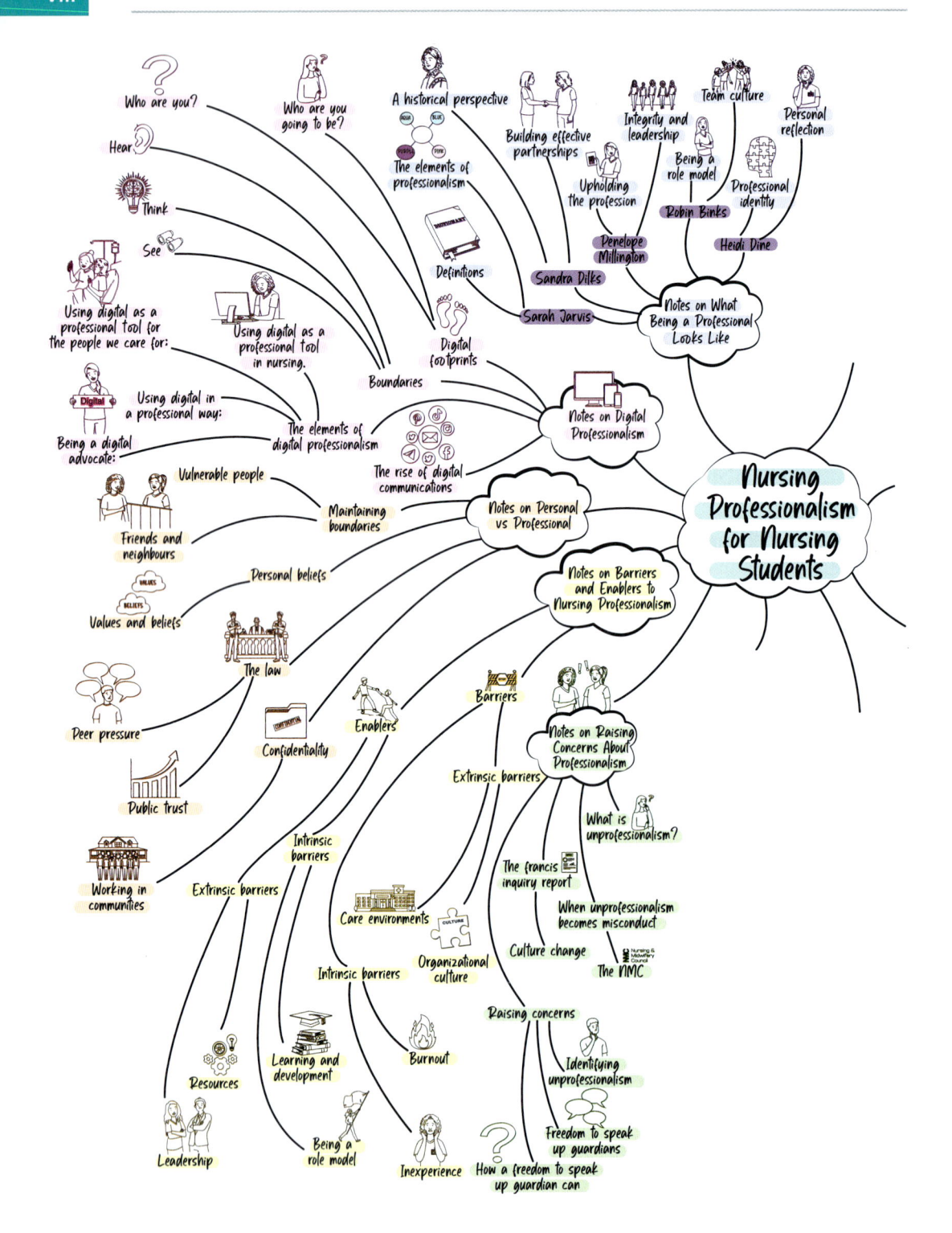

MIND MAP

Nursing Professionalism for Nursing Students

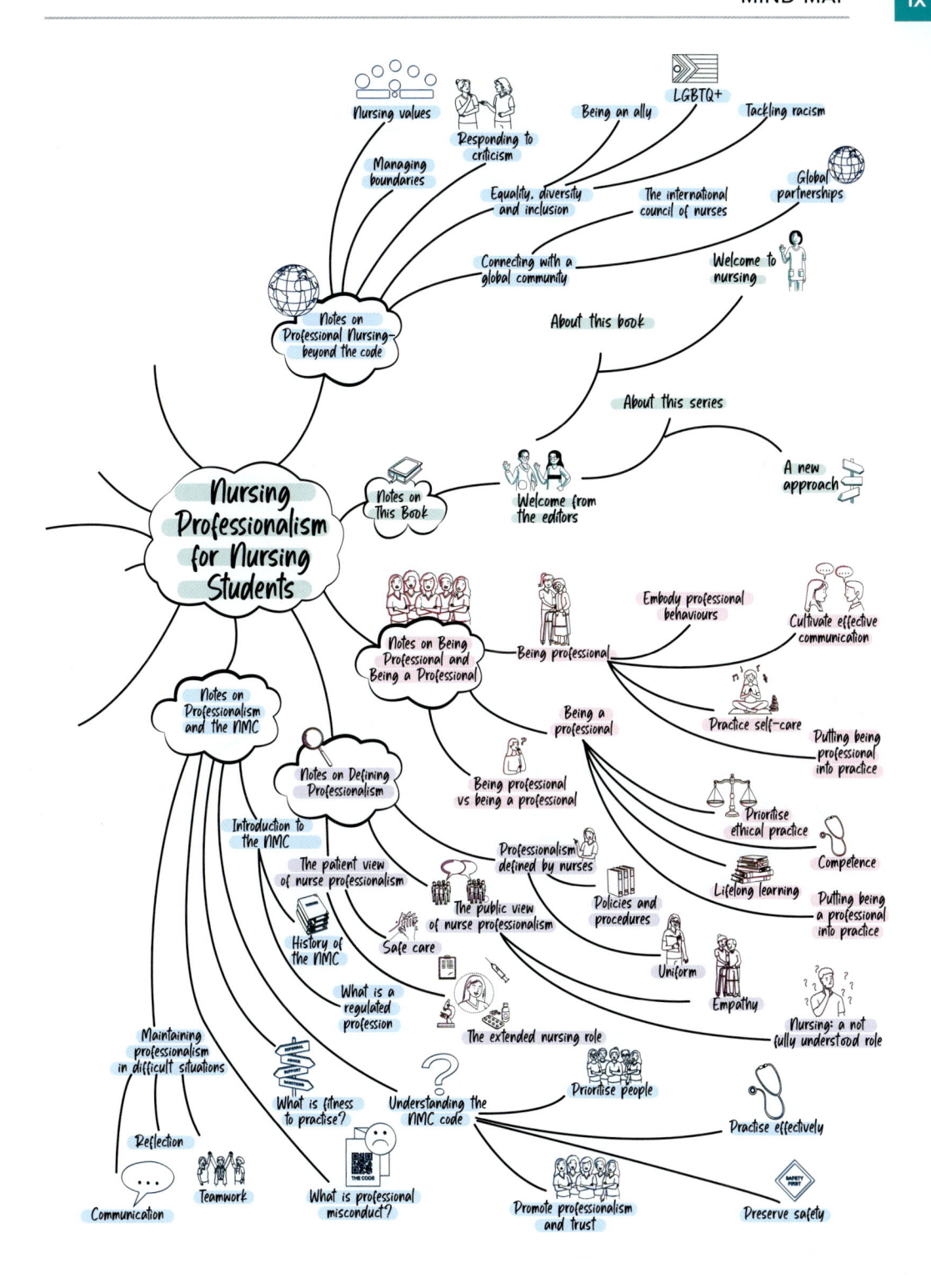

- Notes on Professional Nursing – beyond the code
  - Nursing values
  - Responding to criticism
  - Managing boundaries
  - Being an ally
  - LGBTQ+
  - Tackling racism
  - Equality, diversity and inclusion
  - The international council of nurses
  - Global partnerships
  - Connecting with a global community
  - Welcome to nursing

- Notes on This Book
  - About this book
  - About this series
  - Welcome from the editors
  - A new approach

- Notes on Being Professional and Being a Professional
  - Being professional
    - Embody professional behaviours
    - Cultivate effective communication
    - Practice self-care
    - Putting being professional into practice
  - Being a professional
    - Being professional vs being a professional
    - Prioritise ethical practice
    - Competence
    - Lifelong learning
    - Putting being a professional into practice

- Notes on Defining Professionalism
  - The patient view of nurse professionalism
  - The public view of nurse professionalism
  - Professionalism defined by nurses
  - Policies and procedures
  - Safe care
  - Uniform
  - Empathy
  - What is a regulated profession
  - The extended nursing role
  - Nursing: a not fully understood role

- Notes on Professionalism and the NMC
  - Introduction to the NMC
  - History of the NMC
  - Maintaining professionalism in difficult situations
    - Reflection
    - Communication
    - Teamwork
  - What is fitness to practise?
  - What is professional misconduct?
  - Understanding the NMC code
    - Prioritise people
    - Practise effectively
    - Preserve safety
    - Promote professionalism and trust

Welcome to nursing

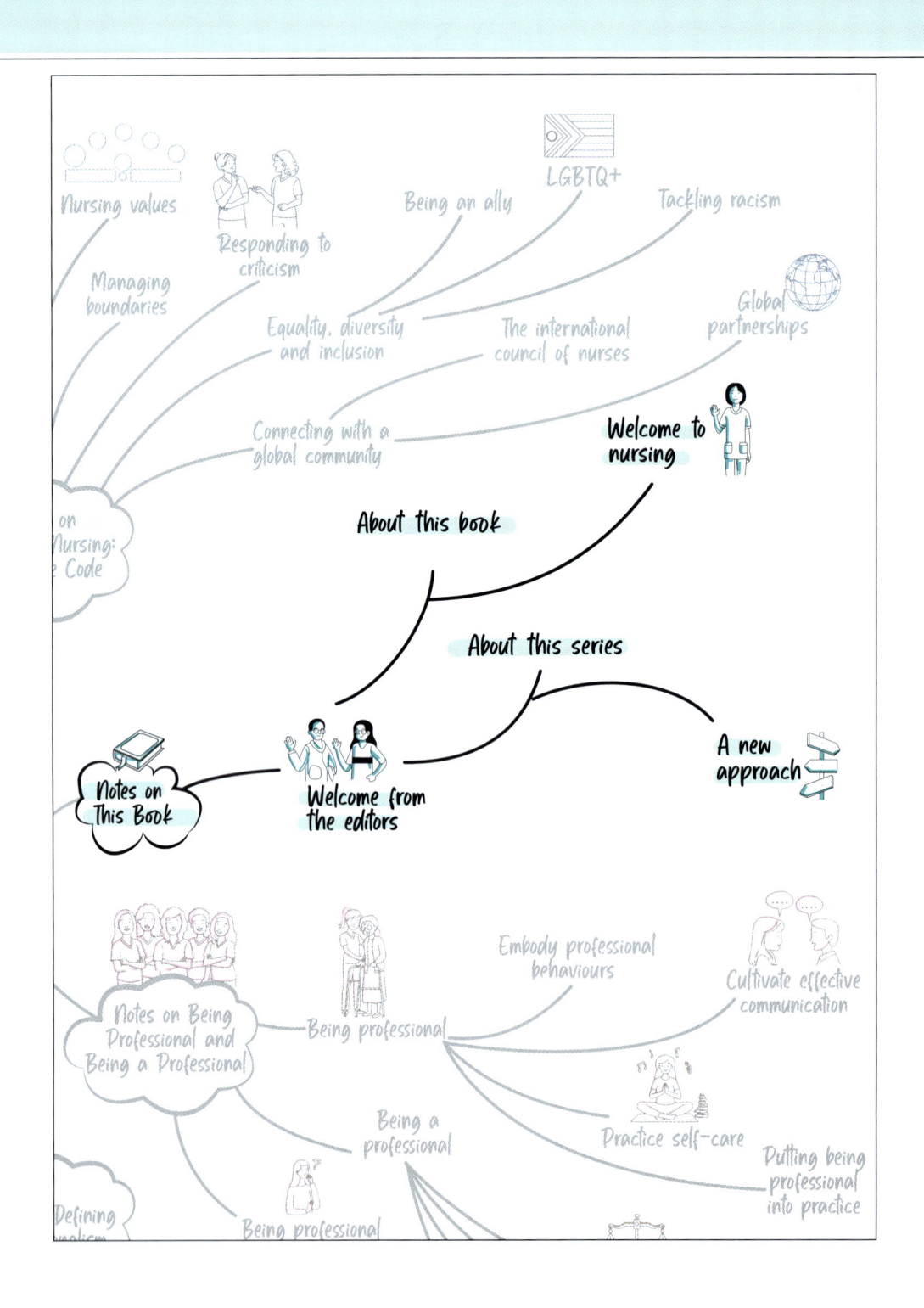

- About this book
  - Notes on This Book
  - Nursing values
  - Managing boundaries
  - Responding to criticism
  - Being an ally
  - LGBTQ+
  - Tackling racism
  - Equality, diversity and inclusion
  - The international council of nurses
  - Global partnerships
  - Connecting with a global community
  - Nursing: The Code

- About this series
  - Welcome from the editors
  - A new approach

- Being professional
  - Notes on Being Professional and Being a Professional
  - Embody professional behaviours
  - Cultivate effective communication
  - Practice self-care
  - Putting being professional into practice
  - Being a professional
  - Defining professionalism
  - Being professional

ABOUT THE SERIES

Teresa Chinn (She/Her) ■ June Girvin (She/Her)

DEAR NURSING STUDENT,

We are so pleased that you have chosen this book from the other nursing books on the shelf! You may have noticed that it looks a little different to other books in the nursing section and there's a very good reason for that – it *is* different! This is the first in a series of books aimed at supporting you as a nursing student. The series combines a nursing book and a digital perspective, including the use of social media, that we hope will create a user-friendly and engaging approach to some of the fundamental topics and challenges in nursing.

The title for the series *New Notes on Nursing* is respectfully and humbly borrowed from Florence Nightingale's own writing. Her *Notes on Nursing* (1860), outlined a vision for health and wellness that encompassed social, political, economic and environmental determinants as well as public health and illness prevention – the bigger picture within which good nursing care must be grounded. We recognise that for many new nursing students, some of the concepts that inform nursing can be challenging and complex, and may not always appear immediately relevant. The *New Notes...* series seeks to address that. We have tried hard to present content in a friendly style, conversational as far as possible, and incorporating social media so that interacting with this book is not a solitary activity but one that can be shared with others who are using the same book and finding out about the same things – whether they are in your cohort or somewhere else in the United Kingdom.

We are trying new design approaches using colourful and engaging content that is aimed at helping you identify the information you need quickly and easily. We understand that sometimes you don't want (or need) to read a dense textbook from start to finish to pull out the most helpful information for your situation, but rather easily identify the bits that are relevant for you at a point in time. We think our colour-coding and infographics throughout the books will help you do just that. We have also included all sorts of helpful 'sidenotes'; again taking inspiration from Florence Nightingale's writing:

THE NMC SAYS
These show the part of the code that the text is relevant to, helping you to embed the code into every area of your practice and thinking.

SOCIAL MEDIA X
'These are tweets from Registered Nurses and nursing students that share snippets of wisdom and perspective'

We have asked many people to contribute to the New Notes on Nursing books and we have included some long quotes from these people; these have been especially written for this series.

CASE STUDY
Case studies, both real and imagined, are a great way to put learning into context, so you will find plenty of them in this series.

ABOUT THE SERIES

> **Your notes are just as important as ours and you will find lots of space in *New Notes on Nursing* for your own notes.**
>
> _____
>
> _____
>
> _____
>
> _____
>
> _____
>
> _____
>
> _____
>
> _____
>
> _____

We have created the books with neurodiversity in mind and have tried to ensure that there is a feeling of space and lightness to the book.

In addition to all of this, we really want to engage and support you on your nursing student journey, so we have created some social media resources for you to tap into. Please search #NewNotesOnNursing and #SuccessfulStN on SOCIAL MEDIA to find out more.

The team of Editors and Authors that we have asked to contribute to *New Notes on Nursing* are all practising health and care professionals, ranging in experience from nursing students and newly qualified Registered Nurses to registered professionals working in clinical and education settings with a wealth of experience. They all wanted to help you. By inviting a variety of voices to create these books, we are sharing many perspectives with you. We hope it helps you to develop well-rounded views on which to start your nursing career.

You are the latest generation of nursing students, and we are so pleased and honoured to be, in some small way, supporting you to flourish. We really hope you enjoy this book (yes, enjoy!) and that, at the end of your student journey, it contains lots of notes scribbled by you, the pages are dog-eared and the cover well-worn – a new generation of nursing texts for a new generation of Registered Nurses.

NURSING PROFESSIONALISM FOR NURSING STUDENTS

Today's nursing is socially complex, politically enmeshed and at times finding its way through conflict and controversy to give the best holistic, person-centred care. We think it's the best career in the world.

Best wishes

June and Teresa

The series is edited by:

> 'I've been a Registered Nurse since 1996 and have made my career in the social care sector. In 2012 set up the nursing Twitter community @WeNurses to help bring together nurses from diverse spheres of practice. I was awarded an MBE for services to nursing in 2014 and in 2018, I was named one of the 70 most influential nurses from 1948 to 2018 by the Royal College of Nursing. I communicate in many different ways in the UK and Europe, particularly on the use of social media in Nursing. I was made a Queens Nurse in 2022'.
>
> **Teresa Chinn, MBE QN @WeNurses**

> 'I qualified as a Registered Nurse in 1976 and have spent a (very) long career in clinical and academic practice. I retired in 2017 and now work independently in roles committed to supporting individual nurses and nursing as a profession – writing, commentating, coaching, reviewing, etc. I was delighted to be asked to support the development of this new series of books and to work with the team of writers/editors and Elsevier'.
>
> **June Girvin @ProfJuneG**

ABOUT THE SERIES

Space for reader's own reflection:

REFERENCES

Nightingale, Florence. 1860. Notes on nursing: what it is, and what it is not. London: Harrison. Harvard (18th ed.).

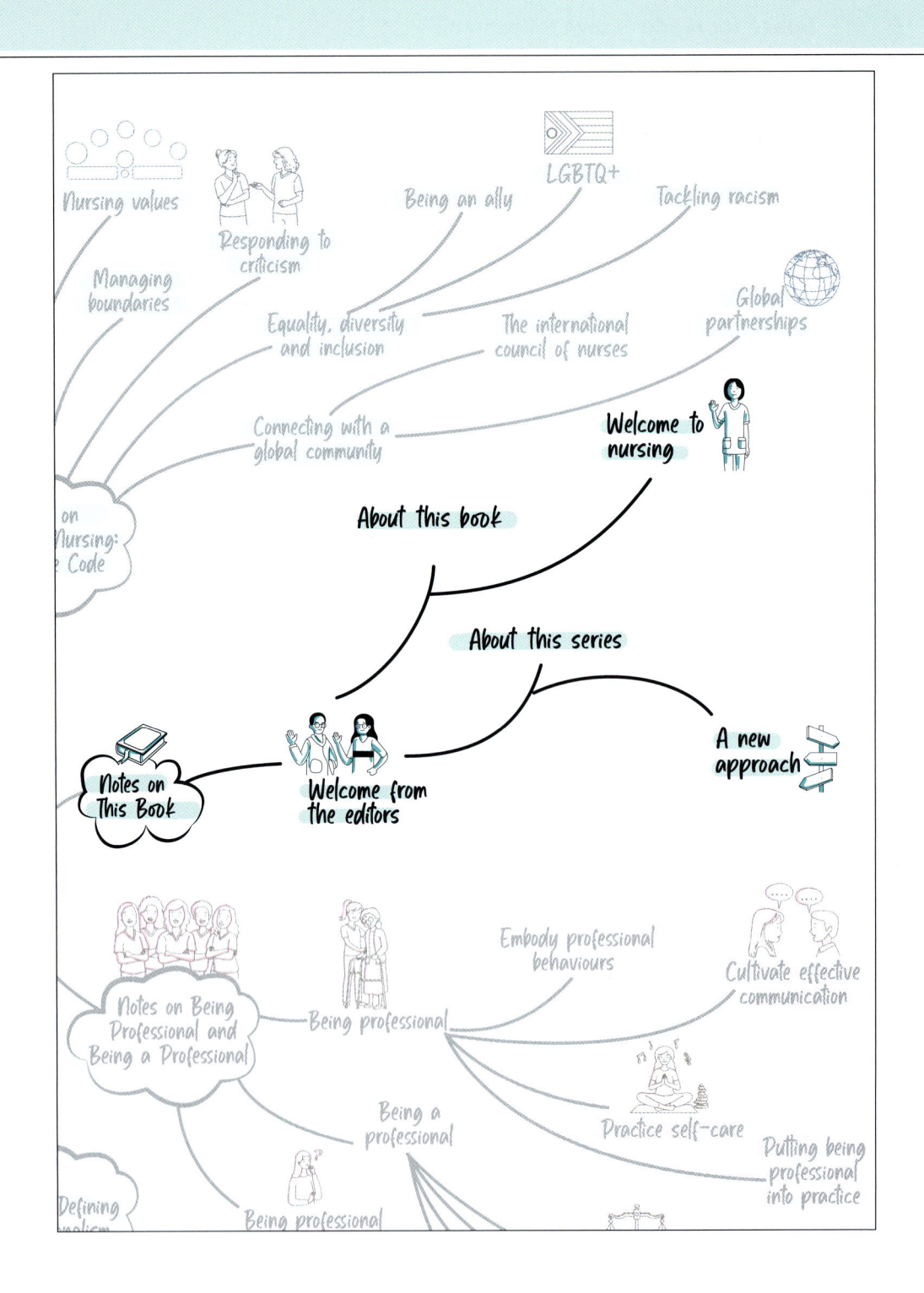

- Nursing values
- Managing boundaries
- Responding to criticism
- Being an ally
- LGBTQ+
- Tackling racism
- Equality, diversity and inclusion
- The international council of nurses
- Global partnerships
- Connecting with a global community
- Welcome to nursing
- About this book
- About this series
- Notes on This Book
- Welcome from the editors
- A new approach
- Notes on Being Professional and Being a Professional
- Being professional
- Embody professional behaviours
- Cultivate effective communication
- Being a professional
- Practice self-care
- Putting being professional into practice
- Defining
- Being professional

ABOUT THIS BOOK

Tara Iles

HELLO, FUTURE NURSES!

Welcome to this book for first-year nursing students. The aim of this book is to enable you to understand some of the topics within nursing and the wider healthcare overview which will be pertinent to you. You will hear from a vast range of expert nurses with various clinical backgrounds and experiences. You will soon realise that one size doesn't fit all, and you will need to use your educational learning and instinct when faced with what can sometimes be challenging situations. That said, if you stay true to your values and periodically remind yourself why you have decided to enter this incredible profession, then you will almost certainly make the right choices in your career.

This book is written by nurses and will read like the nurses are speaking to you. They live and work across the United Kingdom in various settings, from the community to large acute teaching hospital trusts. They will speak to you about their own and others' experiences, what they have learned along the way and, most importantly, from the heart...almost like a diary extract from experienced nurses for you to read. The idea is that you will have the tools to navigate this exciting journey you are embarking on.

So, what is it all about?

This book explores the idea of being a professional and professionalism and all its guises. Firstly, you will hear about the history of nursing as a profession. This chapter is based on a historical context and the development of nursing as a profession. It covers the values associated with nursing and uses scenarios based on the cultural context of nursing. You will then move on to being a professional and understanding more about adhering to the Nursing and Midwifery Council (NMC) code of conduct. You will then hear about professionalism described by various groups of people and what it means to them. How professionalism relates to the NMC code is then explored, which leads to identifying unprofessionalism and how to raise concerns. Interestingly, barriers and enablers to being a professional are discussed as well as how to balance your personal and professional lives, giving some very insightful views. The concept of digital professionalism is also discussed, and what a professional looks like, based on the cultural context of nursing, will be explored. Finally, the wider context is given, that is, global professionalism within nursing.

Professionalism

Professionalism is the skills and competence expected of a profession. Part of being a great nurse is the ability to demonstrate professionalism. A successful nurse, regardless of their title or level, is someone who shows empathy, compassion, credibility and commitment. It is imperative that we commit to personal growth and development and hone our emotional intelligence with time and experience. When we put on our uniform (or ID badge), we have not only a duty of care to our patients and their families and carers but a responsibility to uphold the integrity of our profession. We must remember that people place their trust in us, often at one of the most, if not *the* most, vulnerable times of their lives. We need to assure them that they are right to trust us and that we will always be professional and do what is in the best interests of the patient, regardless of our own beliefs and thoughts.

Expectations of you

As a nursing student, this is your opportunity to witness and participate in real-life scenarios. Be curious, be inquisitive, ask questions and reflect. Remember to be open minded and approach situations as a professional, as a nurse, and ensure all patients have a person-centred approach to their care. Share experiences with your peers, but remember to uphold confidentiality and anonymise scenarios, share best practice and reflect regularly. Remember, self-care should be a high priority for you. We cannot look after others if we do not look after ourselves. Ensure you take a regular break, and seek support when you need it, with whomever you feel most comfortable doing so. Above all, bear in mind that professionalism and the NMC code are core to everything we do as nurses.

> **TIPS**
>
> The following are my tips for achieving everyday professionalism as a nursing student:
>
> - Participate actively in lectures, seminars, skills and simulation sessions. Engage with the learning material to deepen your understanding.
> - Create a study routine that suits your learning style. Break down complex topics, set realistic goals and review regularly.
> - Ask questions. Whether it's in class, during placements or in study groups or tutorials, seeking clarification enhances your comprehension.
> - Connect with fellow nursing students. Form study groups, share experiences and support each other through the ups and downs of the programme.
> - Regularly reflect on your experiences—both in theory and practice learning. Identify areas for improvement, and celebrate successes.
> - Ensure you get enough rest, maintain a healthy lifestyle and seek support when needed.
> - Take advantage of the resources available to you—library materials, online databases and academic support services. They are there to enhance your learning.
> - Keep track of assessments, deadlines and shift patterns. Staying organised will help reduce stress and ensure you meet all your commitments.
> - Attend online webinars, networking events, conferences and career fairs. Building connections with experienced professionals can provide insights and open doors to future opportunities.
> - Acknowledge and celebrate your achievements, whether big or small. Completing assignments, mastering a new skill or successfully completing a placement—every step counts!

Before you start delving into each chapter, use the following space to start to chart your nursing journey:

- Write down your **motivations** for pursuing nursing, the challenges you anticipate and what success in your studies looks like to you.
- Reflect on your **expectations**. Think about personal commitments you are willing to make to meet these expectations, considering dedication and curiosity and embracing challenges.
- Consider creating a visual representation (chart, mind map or timeline) of your **envisioned journey** through the preregistration nursing degree programme. Highlight key milestones, potential challenges and areas where you anticipate personal and professional growth.
- In response to the four elements of **success**—understanding, resilience, reflective practice and community—jot down specific actions or strategies you plan to implement to embody each of these aspects in your academic journey.
- Choose three **tips** from the provided list that resonate most with you, and reflect on how you plan to incorporate these tips into your study routine or daily life as a nursing student.
- Conclude your reflective activity with a brief paragraph summarising your **key takeaways** from this introduction. Consider how this reflective exercise has shaped your mindset as you embark on learning how to be successful in your nursing studies.

_____

_____

_____

_____

Remember, this activity is a personal exploration, and there are no right or wrong answers. It's a tool for self-discovery, goal setting and envisioning your unique journey to becoming a professional.

Some last thoughts from me...

Studying nursing can be challenging physically, emotionally, financially and ethically. Be kind to yourself, and stay true to who you are. Treat people how you would like to be treated, and remember that the standard you walk past is the standard you accept. Find the confidence to speak to someone you trust if you see or hear something that doesn't align with your values or the values of nursing. I don't say this lightly, as I remember very clearly some uncomfortable situations from when I was a student nurse. Thankfully, culture has changed significantly since then, but I remember not having the confidence to share my thoughts, both positive and otherwise, and therefore, I would encourage you to do so. Continuous learning, insight and reflection are key. Nursing and the wider healthcare landscape are evolving and will continue to do so. It's therefore imperative that we, as the largest profession within health and care, are committed to evolving with it. It can, at times, feel overwhelming studying and working practically, but this is the start of an amazing journey for you, with so many opportunities that are so varied. The sky really is the limit, the impact you can and will make. Remember how you feel now: unsure perhaps, maybe some imposter syndrome is creeping in, out of your comfort zone, a bit anxious even. Keep that with you and remember how you feel, as I have done throughout my career. This will empower you. Use it to the best of your ability, as your confidence *will* grow, and remind yourself how you feel now when you are speaking with patients who may have some of these feelings, and with students in the future. You will meet many amazing people from all walks of life, and you will touch their lives, sometimes in ways you may never know or understand. That is the beauty of nursing; we are in an extremely privileged position to comfort people when they are sometimes at their lowest, frightened or panicked. We are the first people to be present when people enter the world and the last when they leave the world. What a responsibility but a huge opportunity to make a real difference and lasting impact.

The best of luck to you with your learning and future careers. I would love to see which paths you choose to follow, so do follow me on X at @tarailes, and use the hashtag #professionalisminnursing. I am keen to hear from you.

Welcome to one of the best clubs in the world...nursing!

Best wishes,
Tara

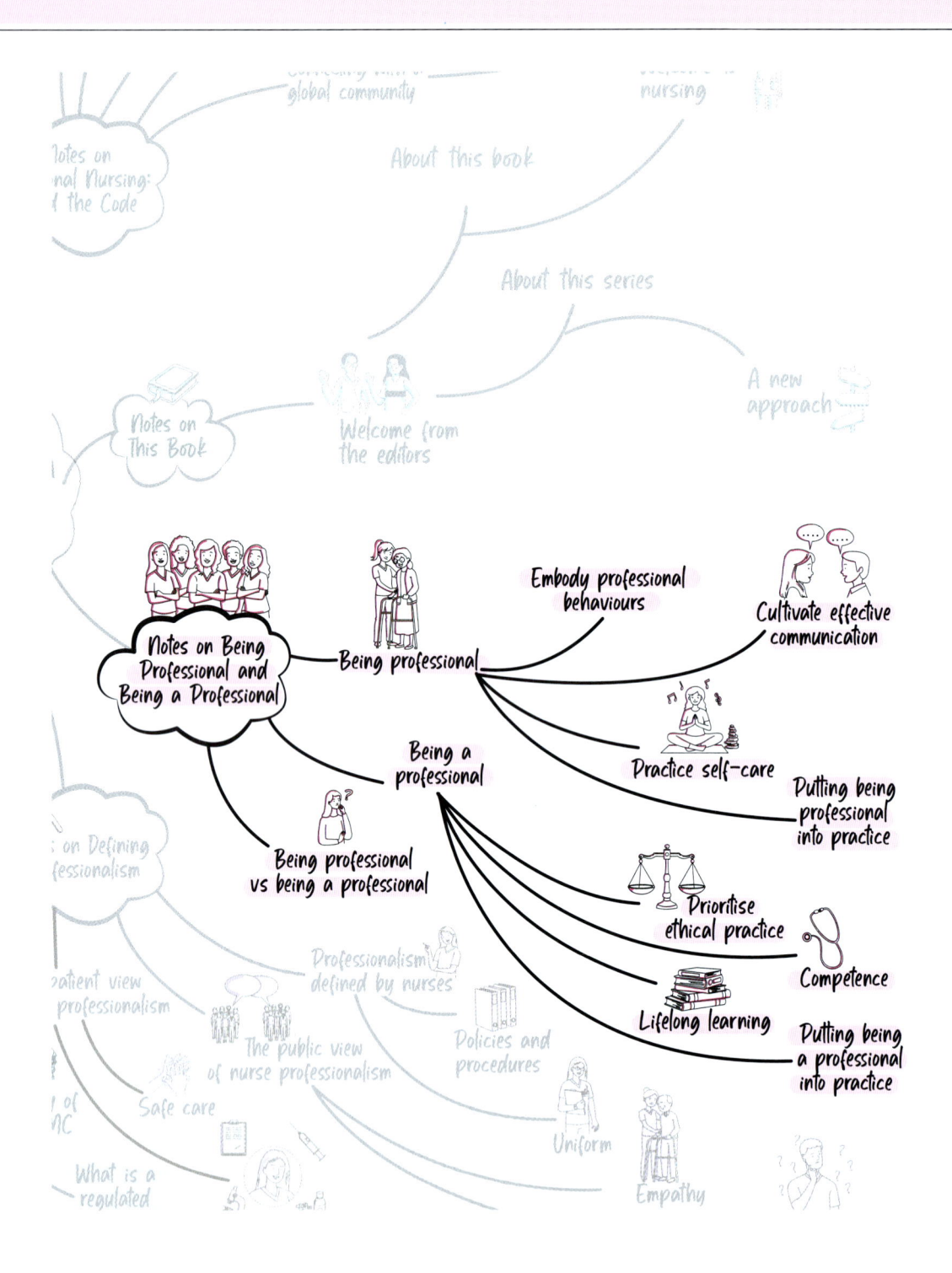

Notes on Being Professional and Being a Professional

- **Being professional**
  - Embody professional behaviours
  - Cultivate effective communication
  - Practice self-care
  - Putting being professional into practice
- **Being a professional**
  - Prioritise ethical practice
  - Competence
  - Lifelong learning
  - Putting being a professional into practice
- **Being professional vs being a professional**

NOTES ON BEING PROFESSIONAL AND BEING A PROFESSIONAL

Nick Browning (he/his)

INTRODUCTION

As a newly qualified nurse, your transition from student to professional practitioner is an exciting and challenging journey. This chapter aims to explore the concept of nursing professionalism and discuss the valuable lessons that can be learned during the early years of your nursing career. Understanding and embodying professionalism is essential for providing high-quality patient care, fostering positive relationships with colleagues and achieving personal growth and fulfilment in your profession.

DEFINING NURSING PROFESSIONALISM

In the context of this chapter, we need to define professionalism in two parts:

- Being professional—Nursing professionalism encompasses a set of values, behaviours and attitudes that guide nurses in their interactions with patients, families and the healthcare team.
- Being a professional—Nurses are bound by the Nursing and Midwifery Council (NMC) code and professional standards. Nurses need to maintain ethical standards, demonstrate competence and exhibit a commitment to lifelong learning and personal development.

Ultimately, professionalism, with its values and behaviours, is intertwined with the NMC's professional standards and provides the foundation upon which nursing practice is built, shaping the way nurses approach their responsibilities and contribute to the healthcare system.

BEING PROFESSIONAL

Embody professional behaviour

Values give a practitioner a base in which to refer when questioning both their own and others' actions and professionalism. Professionalism extends beyond clinical competence and encompasses behaviour, ethics and accountability.

> **THE NMC SAYS**
>
> **20.1** Keep to and uphold the standards and values set out in the Code.

'As a newly qualified nurse, be mindful of your actions, appearance and demeanour. Maintain a professional appearance by adhering to the dress code and practising good personal hygiene. Demonstrate punctuality, reliability and integrity in all aspects of your work. Uphold patient confidentiality and privacy, and respect cultural diversity. Recognise that you are part of a team, and foster a collaborative and respectful work environment'.

> *'I started studying adult nursing in 2012, and from the beginning I found the process challenging, failing to reach anything above 50% in many of my assignments; however, I couldn't have been more excited to hit the shop floor as an adult nurse. I pushed through after a "touch and go" final year, retaking my dissertation. While my final year as a student nurse drew closer, my professional behaviour was tested, where my final year tutor confidently informed me, I should make sure*

1 | NOTES ON BEING PROFESSIONAL AND BEING A PROFESSIONAL

> *I "rationalise" any expectation of going on to further study. At this point, I wanted the world to swallow me up. I had yet to receive the results of my dissertation retake, and my tutor is telling me to rationalise expectations… I was sure I was set to re-do the year, and maybe reconsider my career in nursing. This, on reflection, was lesson one in maintaining an acceptable professional behaviour: "Don't jump to be too emotive on the spot". Take time to process results, comments, and advice; it may be the fuel that ignites your passion and drives you to your goals. I use the word acceptable tactfully, as it leads me to the second lesson I learnt: "it's okay to feel, and be frustrated or even angry with feedback, just make sure your response is acceptable". Being able to accept and understand the truth in healthcare, that is, opinions become a large part of the working world. Opinions in a collective can be incredibly powerful; joining informed opinion with a good evidence base creates a solid foundation for exceptional care. Opinions in isolation, however, can be destructive and separating. Take time to work out which is which, and form your own, but remember to do so carefully, and support them with some solid evidence. These initial comments will give a grounding to ensure you are acting as a professional, with integrity, allowing your behaviours to follow in the same trend.*
>
> *Nick Browning, Trust Lead for Advanced Practice*

Attitudes

Attitudes in nursing are the bedrock of compassionate and effective patient care. They shape the overall patient experience, impacting not just medical outcomes but emotional well-being. A nurse's attitude sets the tone for trust, comfort and communication, crucial elements in fostering a healing environment. Empathy, patience and respect exhibited through attitudes provide a sense of understanding and support, easing anxieties and empowering patients in their healthcare journey. Alongside this, positive attitudes among nurses and other allied health professionals create a collaborative and harmonious work environment that directly translates to better patient care. An interesting literature review by Ryan (2016) explored nursing students' attitudes towards evidence-based practice (EBP) and found that whilst evidence points towards nursing students generally having a positive attitude towards EBP, there are many things that affect that attitude, including the practical aspects of nursing taking over, culture, confidence in ability, role models and clinical support. Attitudes in nursing are the invisible threads that weave together competence and compassion, ultimately defining the quality of care provided.

> **SOCIAL MEDIA X**
> @PUNCabz
>
> What makes a professional? Have a positive attitude. Provide quality care. Challenge decisions when necessary. Respect boundaries. Accept responsibility. Remember those 6 C's & 4 P's!

> **SOCIAL MEDIA X**
> @MaryDunningTU
>
> remembering we are the culture, we are the profession, believe a professional attitude is key, responding respectfully. Being mindful of past, present and future. Asking ourselves Enabling professional today, what will you do...lead by example.

Cultivate effective communication

Effective communication is a cornerstone of nursing professionalism. As a nurse, you will interact with patients, families and a diverse healthcare team on a daily basis. Balzer-Riley (2017) explores communication in nursing by stating:

- 'communication is a lifelong journey;
- you can make a difference in patients' lives by practicing caring, assertive, responsible communication;

1 | NOTES ON BEING PROFESSIONAL AND BEING A PROFESSIONAL

- as you grow in comfort with assertive skills, you will build positive relationships in your professional and personal life;
- you support each other's rights for ethical, competent, caring practice as you have the courage to grow your own assertive communication skills;
- you make a difference even in short moments of connection and that you always have enough time as you learn how to be fully present'.

Being able to communicate clearly, effectively and compassionately is a key skill for all nursing students and a huge part of being professional. The NMC Code succinctly sets out expectations in regard to communication:

> **THE NMC SAYS**
>
> 7 Communicate clearly. To achieve this, you must:
>   7.1 Use terms that people in your care, colleagues and the public can understand.
>   7.2 Take reasonable steps to meet people's language and communication needs, providing, wherever possible, assistance to those who need help to communicate their own or other people's needs.
>   7.3 Use a range of verbal and non-verbal communication methods, and consider cultural sensitivities, to better understand and respond to people's personal and health needs.
>   7.4 Check people's understanding from time to time to keep misunderstanding or mistakes to a minimum.
>   7.5 Be able to communicate clearly and effectively in English.

Developing strong communication skills will enable you to establish therapeutic relationships, promote patient-centred care and collaborate effectively with colleagues. Active listening, empathy and clarity in conveying information are crucial aspects of communication that should be cultivated early in your career.

Active listening—Being an active listener is about being engaged in receiving and decoding the messages that patients send. This involves not only listening to the verbal content of what the patient is saying but also observing nonverbal communication and using this to assess their current emotional state (Gault et al. 2017).

> **TIPS**
>
> Miller (2023) identifies five tips for active listening:
>
> '1. Ensure you have undisturbed, confidential time to be with the patient
> 2. Be fully present – practise focusing and not being distracted by your own thoughts and reactions or by noises and other people around you
> 3. Look at the patient and listen to what they are saying
> 4. Be aware of nonverbal communication, for example, signs that may suggest confusion or anxiety. Then check with the patient to see if that is what they are feeling
> 5. Ensure you have clinical supervision to support you when working with patients experiencing trauma – and use it to develop your skills'.

Empathy—Empathy is a key skill to develop in nursing. Brown (2013) created a renowned YouTube video around empathy where she describes empathy as fuelling connection, recognising another person's perspective, being nonjudgemental and recognising emotion in other people and communicating that. She states that ultimately empathy is feeling *with* people.

> **TIPS**
>
> Norwich University (n.d.) has some great tips around incorporating empathy into nursing practice:
>
> 1. Listen to patients and show curiosity about their lives
> 2. Be kind and respectful
> 3. Develop cultural competence and awareness
> 4. Use self-care strategies to prevent compassion fatigue
> 5. Lead by example.

1 | NOTES ON BEING PROFESSIONAL AND BEING A PROFESSIONAL

Clarity—Clear communication that is unambiguous and to the point is vital, as often nurses communicate in highly stressful situations that require communication to be certain. Clarity is also important when communicating with people who have communication difficulties, for example, someone who has hearing loss or someone with dementia.

> **TIPS**
>
> A great way to develop clarity in communication is to practice SBAR handovers (NHS England & NHS Improvement 2022):
>
> 'Situation: I am (name), (X) nurse on ward (X) I am calling about (patient X) I am calling because I am concerned that… (e.g., BP is low/high, pulse is XX, temperature is XX, early warning score is XX).
>
> Background: Patient (X) was admitted on (XX date) with… (e.g., myocardial infarction/chest infection) They have had (X operation/procedure/investigation) Patient (X)'s condition has changed in the last (XX mins) Their last set of obs were (XX) Patient (X)'s normal condition is… (e.g., alert/drowsy/confused, pain free).
>
> Assessment: I think the problem is (XXX) And I have… (e.g., given O_2/analgesia, stopped the infusion) OR I am not sure what the problem is but patient (X) is deteriorating OR I don't know what's wrong but I am really worried.
>
> Recommendation: need you to… Come to see the patient in the next (XX mins) AND Is there anything I need to do in the meantime? (e.g., stop the fluid/repeat the obs)'.

Recognise the power of your words and strive to communicate respectfully and compassionately, even in challenging situations.

> 'As a nurse, I believe communication is the heartbeat of quality care. It's not just about relaying information; it's the cornerstone of trust, comfort, and healing. Clear and empathetic communication fosters connections with patients, easing fears, and creates a space where patients feel heard and understood, as well as colleagues. It's not merely about the words spoken but the manner in which they're delivered—gentle reassurances during moments of uncertainty or clear instructions that empower patients to take charge of their health. Effective communication isn't a luxury; it's an essential tool that builds bridges between medical expertise and a patient's journey toward wellness'.
>
> **Nick Browning, Trust Lead for Advanced Practice**

Practice self-care

Nursing can be physically and emotionally demanding. To provide optimal care for others, you must prioritise self-care. Recognise the signs of burnout and compassion fatigue and take steps to prevent them. Engage in activities that promote your well-being, such as exercise, hobbies, spending time with loved ones and seeking support from a mentor or counsellor. Remember that self-care is not selfish but essential for maintaining your own professional standards.

THE NMC SAYS

20.9 Maintain the level of health you need to carry out your professional role.

Smart and Creighton (2022) state that nursing students 'should take responsibility for their own wellbeing to ensure continued safe practice. Practising self-care is a great first step'.

1 | NOTES ON BEING PROFESSIONAL AND BEING A PROFESSIONAL

> **TIPS**
>
> Try this mindfulness activity as part of your self-care (Smart and Creighton 2022):
>
> 'Close your eyes, breathe in deeply for a count of five and breathe out for five. Repeat three times. Open your eyes and identify the following:
> - Five things you can see
> - Four things you can reach out to and touch
> - Three sounds you can hear
> - Two things you can smell
> - One thing you can taste'.

Self-care doesn't have to be mindfulness; however, it can be anything that helps you to recharge:

- Exercise
- Eating well
- Chilling in front of the TV
- Reading
- Taking a long bath
- Listening to music
- Yoga
- Taking regular breaks from work
- Deep breathing
- Meditation
- Petting your dog...or cat

How do you practice self-care, and how will you ensure you make time to do this over your nursing career:

_____
_____
_____
_____
_____

Putting 'being professional' into practice

In nursing practice, being a professional encompasses a multifaceted approach that embodies expertise, ethics, compassion and continuous learning. It involves upholding high standards of care, adhering to ethical principles and demonstrating competence in clinical skills and decision making. Putting this into practice extends beyond technical proficiency; it encompasses integrity, respect and advocacy for patients' rights and well-being. It involves effective communication within interdisciplinary teams, maintaining confidentiality and continually updating knowledge to provide evidence-based care. Being a professional in nursing means embracing a commitment to lifelong learning, adapting to advancements in healthcare and continuously striving for excellence while putting the patient's needs at the forefront of every decision and action.

> *'It's important to remember that every team has its challenges, every colleague has a bad day, and you, too, will have days you question your career choice. Remember that those around you will likely feed off your emotions as much as you feed off theirs. Try to give time to those who need it, remembering to reserve energy for yourself. Being a staff nurse is no underrated position. You will find yourself guiding a workforce who will look to you for guidance, reassurance, and, a lot of the time, ownership of clinical scenarios. You need to have the energy to give to a number of people, so be cautious of giving too much and burning out.*
>
> *Within my first year, I found establishing myself amongst my peer staff nurses and the healthcare assistant (HCA) workforce difficult. It was as if the two sets of professionals were at odds. If I took too long to perform the medication round or put up the morning IVs, then I felt I was letting the HCAs down. If I prioritised washes and breakfast I was falling back on my staff nurse medical duties. It was a hard balance. On reflection, one core tip would be to manage expectations early. Make a plan with the HCA at the start of the shift, act as a team and break down any "hierarchy". We are all here for the same reason; we just have different roles. If you make your plan together, it will show*

authentic teamwork, inclusivity and allow your teammate to understand your other duties and responsibilities, which is likely to lead them to giving you an easier time, especially early in your career!

As I progressed through the year, I noticed that my professionalism was tested. There were scenarios where colleagues would comment on the cleanliness of a patient and say they "didn't want to go in to do a wash", or that they "needed a nose clip to go in". I felt in some ways a pressure to join in, to be on the team, to not be boring, or testing. I found myself in a place I didn't want to be, between my patients and my team. I remember going back to the senior nurse of the ward and asking how to address these comments and being met with a lack of advice, to put it nicely. A big thing to remember is nursing isn't everything, and the chances are, your friends and family outside of work have almost certainly been through the same processes and scenarios in their workplaces. If you feel unable to offload to your colleagues, seek it from your other networks; you will be amazed how much will overlap, and how much peace you can source from just talking it through. The NMC Code of Conduct (2018) states we must always respect a patient's dignity, privacy, and autonomy. So, if you feel any of these are compromised, even by small comments, then seek advice in and out of work on strategies to dissolve that risk. Sometimes, you just have to say, "that's enough now guys, let's get on", and people will listen, and almost always respect the assertive, advocating tone.

Progressing through the year posed an ongoing challenge professionally. I wanted to strive to take opportunities, but also "earn my stripes" in the role. I recall being encouraged by the senior staff nurse on the ward to take charge as an acting nurse in charge, while being told by others to make the most of being a staff nurse with set patients. This posed my first progression challenge, setting boundaries and being true to what you want. It is okay to take opportunity where others have not been offered. You may feel, as you progress into your formative years, that taking opportunity where others have not been offered is seen as selfish, or greedy.

Continued

The chances are, if someone puts you forward or encourages you do to something, then you are ready! When you're taking such opportunity, remain composed, factual and a bit proud; it's likely to inspire others to push for notice, recognition and opportunity. This phase in your career is about leading by example, even early on. Once I had performed a few months in charge, a band 6 charge nurse role came up. I didn't know what to do. I had been constantly reminded that the role required more years in the game, more hours, more experience, more wards worked. What I knew is that GI surgical was my area, an area I knew I wanted to progress in, even though at the time I didn't know exactly what this looked like. After some comments saying it was too early, and a bit of reluctance on my side, I applied! Preparation will demonstrate how serious you are about any role. You will have prepared relentlessly to be a student nurse; don't stop that drive in your career. I prepared extensively, talking to everyone I could about the role, and gained insight into what I could offer other members of the team. When progressing in any direction in your career, seek attention and advice from other professions; you will be surprised how much our roles overlap and how the nursing profession acts as a stabiliser in any ward, outpatient and community environment'.

Nick Browning, Trust Lead for Advanced Practice

CASE STUDY

Being a professional in practice: self-care of the student nurse

Beth, a third-year student nurse, has been working in a busy hospital's emergency department for her 8-week placement. She has been known for her exceptional dedication and empathy towards patients, and she often finds herself working long shifts, frequently sacrificing breaks to ensure her patients receive the best care possible. However, lately, Beth has been feeling increasingly fatigued, emotionally drained and struggling with insomnia.

> **CASE STUDY—cont'd**
>
> Despite her passion for nursing, Beth's self-care has taken a backseat. Her routine lacks proper nutrition and exercise, and she often feels guilty about taking time off or prioritising her own well-being over her patients. She finds it challenging to set boundaries.
>
> Beth's colleagues, and particularly her mentor, have noticed the changes in her demeanour and have expressed concern about her well-being. Recognising her passion for nursing but also the importance of self-care, they encourage Beth to attend workshops on stress management and self-care techniques via the university. They emphasise the significance of setting boundaries, utilising available resources for support and practising mindfulness techniques to alleviate the emotional burden of caring for critically ill patients.
>
> Despite initial hesitation, Beth begins to attend these workshops and gradually incorporates small self-care practices into her routine. She starts setting boundaries regarding her work hours, prioritising breaks for meals and rest, and engaging in regular exercise. She also begins to confide in her colleagues and seeks guidance from a mentor, allowing her to process the emotional challenges that come with nursing.
>
> Over time, Beth notices significant improvements in her well-being. She feels more energised during her shifts, experiences improved sleep patterns and feels more emotionally resilient when faced with challenging situations in the emergency department. By prioritising self-care, Beth not only enhances her own health but also becomes a more effective and compassionate nurse, capable of providing higher-quality care to her patients.

This case study underscores the importance of nurses recognising the need for self-care within their demanding profession. Balancing dedication to patient care with personal well-being is crucial for sustaining a fulfilling and effective nursing practice. It highlights the significance of establishing healthy boundaries, seeking support from colleagues and embracing self-care strategies to maintain both physical and emotional health in the demanding field of nursing.

> ✏️ **Think about what self-care looks like for you and how it can help you with being professional:**
>
> _____
>
> _____
>
> _____
>
> _____

BEING A PROFESSIONAL

The NMC Code of Practice is the ethical framework that guides nursing practice, emphasising professionalism at its core. It articulates the values, behaviours and standards expected of nurses in the United Kingdom. Adherence to this code is fundamental in defining professionalism in nursing. It underscores the importance of delivering high-quality care while upholding integrity, compassion and respect for individuals' dignity and rights. The code directs nurses to prioritise patient well-being, promote autonomy and maintain confidentiality. It also emphasises the significance of continuous learning, accountability and effective communication within multidisciplinary teams. Ultimately, the NMC Code of Practice serves as a compass, shaping nurses' conduct and decisions, thereby reinforcing and defining the essence of professionalism within the nursing profession.

Prioritise ethical practice

Ethical dilemmas are an inevitable part of nursing practice. Early in your career, you will encounter situations where you must make difficult decisions that align with your professional values and ethical principles. It is essential to develop a strong ethical framework and the ability to critically analyse ethical issues. Familiarise yourself with the nursing code of ethics and seek guidance from experienced mentors or ethics committees when faced with moral challenges. Upholding ethical standards builds trust with patients, colleagues and the broader healthcare community.

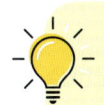

TIPS

Tips on being professional in practice

- Keep a check on eye contact: It will show your engagement. Furthermore, if you're listening, keep eye contact; if you're talking, you can break eye contact as a rule (Davidhizar, 1992). Adhere to ethical standards; uphold the ethical principles outlined in the nursing code of conduct (NMC Code of Conduct, 2015). Respect patient confidentiality, advocate for their rights and prioritise their well-being.
- Continuous learning: Embrace a lifelong learning attitude. Stay updated with the latest medical advancements, attend training sessions and pursue further education to enhance skills and knowledge.
- Effective communication: Develop strong communication skills. Listen actively, convey information clearly and collaborate effectively within the healthcare team to ensure coordinated patient care.
- Maintain boundaries: Establish clear boundaries between personal and professional life. Learn to say no when necessary, manage workload effectively and prioritise self-care to prevent burnout.
- Cultural sensitivity: Respect diverse cultural backgrounds and beliefs of patients. Cultivate an understanding and appreciation for cultural differences to provide culturally competent care.
- Empathy and compassion: Demonstrate empathy and compassion in interactions with patients. Show understanding and provide emotional support, acknowledging their feelings and concerns.
- Accountability: Take responsibility for your actions and decisions. Be accountable for the care provided, learn from mistakes and strive for improvement.
- Teamwork and collaboration: Foster a collaborative environment within the healthcare team. Value the expertise of others, communicate effectively and work together for optimal patient outcomes.
- Professional appearance and conduct: Maintain a professional appearance and demeanour. Dress appropriately, exhibit professionalism in your behaviour and act as a role model for ethical conduct.
- Self-reflection: Engage in self-reflection to evaluate and improve your practice. Regularly assess your strengths, weaknesses and areas for development to enhance patient care.
- By integrating these tips into daily nursing practice, one can uphold professionalism while delivering high-quality and compassionate care to patients.

Competence

Competence in nursing stands at the heart of delivering safe, effective and high-quality patient care. It encompasses a nurse's ability to merge theoretical knowledge with practical skills, critical thinking and decision making in diverse healthcare settings. Beyond mastering technical expertise, competence involves adaptability to evolving medical advancements and navigating complex situations with confidence and efficiency. Competent nurses not only administer treatments but also anticipate and mitigate potential risks, ensuring patient safety at every step. Their proficiency fosters trust among patients, colleagues and the healthcare community, forming the bedrock of a robust healthcare system. Ultimately, competence in nursing isn't merely about meeting standards; it's about continuously striving for excellence to positively impact patient outcomes and elevate the standard of care within the profession.

Lifelong learning

As a nurse, one of the most important lessons to learn is the value of continuous learning.

> **THE NMC SAYS**
>
> 22.3 Keep your knowledge and skills up to date, taking part in appropriate and regular learning and professional development activities that aim to maintain and develop your competence and improve your performance.

Nursing is a dynamic profession that is constantly evolving, with new research, technologies and EBPs emerging regularly. Embrace opportunities for professional development, attend conferences, pursue advanced certifications and engage in ongoing education to stay current and provide the best possible care to your patients. By adopting a growth mindset and seeking out learning experiences, you will enhance your knowledge, skills and confidence as a nurse.

1 | NOTES ON BEING PROFESSIONAL AND BEING A PROFESSIONAL

CASE STUDY

Sam is a dedicated nurse with 5 years of experience working in a general surgical ward in a hospital. Despite her extensive experience, Sam acknowledges the importance of lifelong learning in nursing. Recently, she encountered a case involving a rare surgical condition that she hadn't encountered before. Although she provided excellent care, Sam realised there were gaps in her knowledge about this specific condition and its treatment.

Although Sam initially felt disheartened, she saw this as an opportunity for growth. She actively sought out resources and participated in online seminars, connecting with specialists in the field. Sam delved into recent research articles and consulted with her colleagues to gain a comprehensive understanding of the condition.

Through her dedication to learning, Sam not only expanded her knowledge about the rare surgical condition but also developed a deeper insight into various treatment modalities. This not only benefited her patient but also enhanced Sam's overall practice as a nurse. She now regularly shares her newfound knowledge with her team, contributing to ongoing discussions and initiatives aimed at improving patient care within her unit.

Sam's commitment to lifelong learning not only enriched her professional expertise but also reinforced the importance of continuously seeking knowledge and skill enhancement in the dynamic field of nursing.

What are your thoughts about the importance of lifelong learning?

_____
_____
_____
_____
_____

Putting 'being a professional' to practise

Although being a nursing student can feel frustrating, lonely and never ending, don't worry—it does get better! Hopefully while you are on this journey you can reflect on the amazing, unlimited and rewarding experiences it has to offer. It's important to acknowledge that when you qualify as a nurse, you are an immense resource to the organisation, your future team and the patients and families you will have contact with.

> **CASE STUDY**
>
> Max is a seasoned nurse who worked in an oncology unit and cared for Mr. Adams, a middle-aged man diagnosed with advanced-stage cancer. Despite a poor prognosis, Mr. Adams adamantly refused further potentially life-prolonging chemotherapy treatment, stating concern with the side effects and his desire to avoid prolonging what he perceived as inevitable suffering.
>
> Understanding the balance of Mr. Adams's choice and respecting his decision, Max engaged in a professional and empathetic approach. He spent time listening to his concerns, validating his emotions and acknowledging the complexity of his decision. Max used his communication skills, using gentle persuasion to encourage Mr. Adams to reconsider treatment, highlighting potential benefits while acknowledging his fears and concerns.
>
> Max was aware of maintaining the therapeutic relationship he had built and ensured that Mr. Adams felt listened to and respected. Max provided evidence-based knowledge to support Mr. Adams in making a truly informed decision, establishing trust.
>
> Max worked with the healthcare team to explore alternative options and supportive care measures that aligned with Mr. Adams's wishes. With this, Max worked with Mr. Adams to engage with the palliative care services, pain management strategies and psychological support teams to ensure Mr. Adams received comprehensive care despite his refusal of conventional treatment. With this, Mr. Adams felt supported in his care episode and felt able to confide in Max as an advocate. Max's approach highlights the essence of professionalism in nursing care and the robust relationship that can be established with trust, empathy and respect for choices.

It is clear that nursing professionalism extends beyond detecting the deteriorating patient and administering treatment. It focuses on the attitude, respecting patients and their wishes, even when we as practitioners don't necessarily agree, and exploring with the patient other options and alternative treatments.

BEING PROFESSIONAL VERSUS BEING A PROFESSIONAL

Sometimes our professional code of conduct conflicts with 'being a professional'. There are occasions where decisions must be made in the 'patient's best interest'. This is often the case where patients lack capacity to make a well-informed decision and can be apparent in a range of settings and scenarios. The following is a case study to illuminate this conflict.

> **CASE STUDY**
>
> John, a registered nurse in a psychiatric unit, encountered a patient named Alex, who had a history of bipolar disorder and was admitted due to a severe manic episode. During the assessment, Alex categorically refused medication, stating that it is harmful and will make him more unwell.
>
> John noticed signs of escalating agitation and identified a risk to both Alex and his colleagues, as well as other residents. Knowing the urgency of the situation and assessing the potential risks, John knew that administering the prescribed medication was crucial to prevent harm and stabilise Alex's condition.
>
> Johns' ethical standards and professional responsibilities allowed him to engage in a respectful conversation with Alex, explaining the potential consequences of refusing treatment and the benefits of the prescribed medication in managing the manic episode. However, Alex remained resistant.

Continued

> **CASE STUDY—cont'd**
>
> Considering Alex's compromised capacity due to the acute episode and the imminent risk of harm to those around him, John rapidly consulted his colleagues to gain a consensus on how to proceed, following his local and national protocols. With Alex's best interest in mind, John made the decision to initiate a restraint hold which legally allowed the administration of necessary medication to stabilise Alex's condition and ensure their safety.
>
> Despite initial resistance and distress, Alex's condition gradually improved after receiving the prescribed treatment. As Alex regained stability, they expressed gratitude to John for taking action in their best interest during a period when they were unable to make sound decisions due to their mental health condition.

This example illustrates a situation where a nurse, in adherence to professional ethics and responsibilities, acted in the patient's best interest despite the patient's refusal of treatment. It underscores the importance of balancing patient autonomy with the duty to prevent harm and ensure the overall well-being of the individual under care.

CONCLUSION

When exploring nursing professionalism, it's evident that the essence of nursing extends far beyond technical skills and medical knowledge. Professionalism in nursing encapsulates a multifaceted commitment to ethical conduct, lifelong learning, compassionate care and unwavering dedication to patients' well-being. It's the fusion of empathy, integrity, effective communication and the relentless pursuit of excellence that defines a professional nurse. Embracing this ethos empowers nurses to navigate complex healthcare landscapes, advocate for patients' rights and contribute significantly to the advancement of healthcare. As nursing evolves among societal changes and technological advancements, the foundation of professionalism remains at the core, guiding nurses to uphold the highest standards of care, fostering trust and ensuring the delivery of holistic, patient-centred nursing practice.

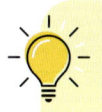

1 | NOTES ON BEING PROFESSIONAL AND BEING A PROFESSIONAL

> **TIPS**
> Remember, have fun. Work is only a part of your life; however, we tend to spend a long time doing it, so enjoy it.

Space for reader's own reflection:
_____
_____
_____
_____
_____

REFERENCES

Balzer-Riley, J., 2017. Communication in nursing, eighth ed. Elsevier, Missouri.

Brown, B., 2013. Brene Brown on empathy. https://www.youtube.com/watch?v=1Evwgu369Jw [Accessed January 18, 2023]

Davidhizar, R., 1992. Interpersonal communication: A review of eye contact. Infect. Control Hosp. Epidemiol. 13 (4), 222–225.

Gault, I., Shapcott, J., Luthi, A., Reid, G., 2017. Communication in nursing and healthcare: A Guide for Compassionate Practice. SAGE, Los Angeles.

Miller, N., 2023. What is active listening and how can I use it? Good communication is essential for effective care and active listening can improve patient outcomes. Nurs. Older People 35 (4), 15–16.

NHS Improvement and NHS England, 2022. SBAR Communication Tool [online]. https://www.england.nhs.uk/wp-content/uploads/2021/03/qsir-sbar-communication-tool.pdf [Accessed January 18, 2024]

NMC. 2015. The NMC Code of Conduct [Online]. NMC. https://www.nmc.org.uk/standards/code/read-the-code-online/ [Accessed July 18, 2023]

Norwich University. n.d. Importance of Empathy in Nursing: 5 Patient Care Tips. https://online.norwich.edu/importance-empathy-nursing-5-patient-care-tips [Accessed January 18, 2024]

Ryan, E., 2016. Undergraduate nursing students' attitudes and use of research and evidence-based practice – an integrative literature review. J. Clin. Nurs. 25 (11-12), 1548–1556.

Smart, A., Creighton, L., 2022. Professionalism in nursing 3: The value of self-care for students. Nurs. Times 118 (6), 45–47.

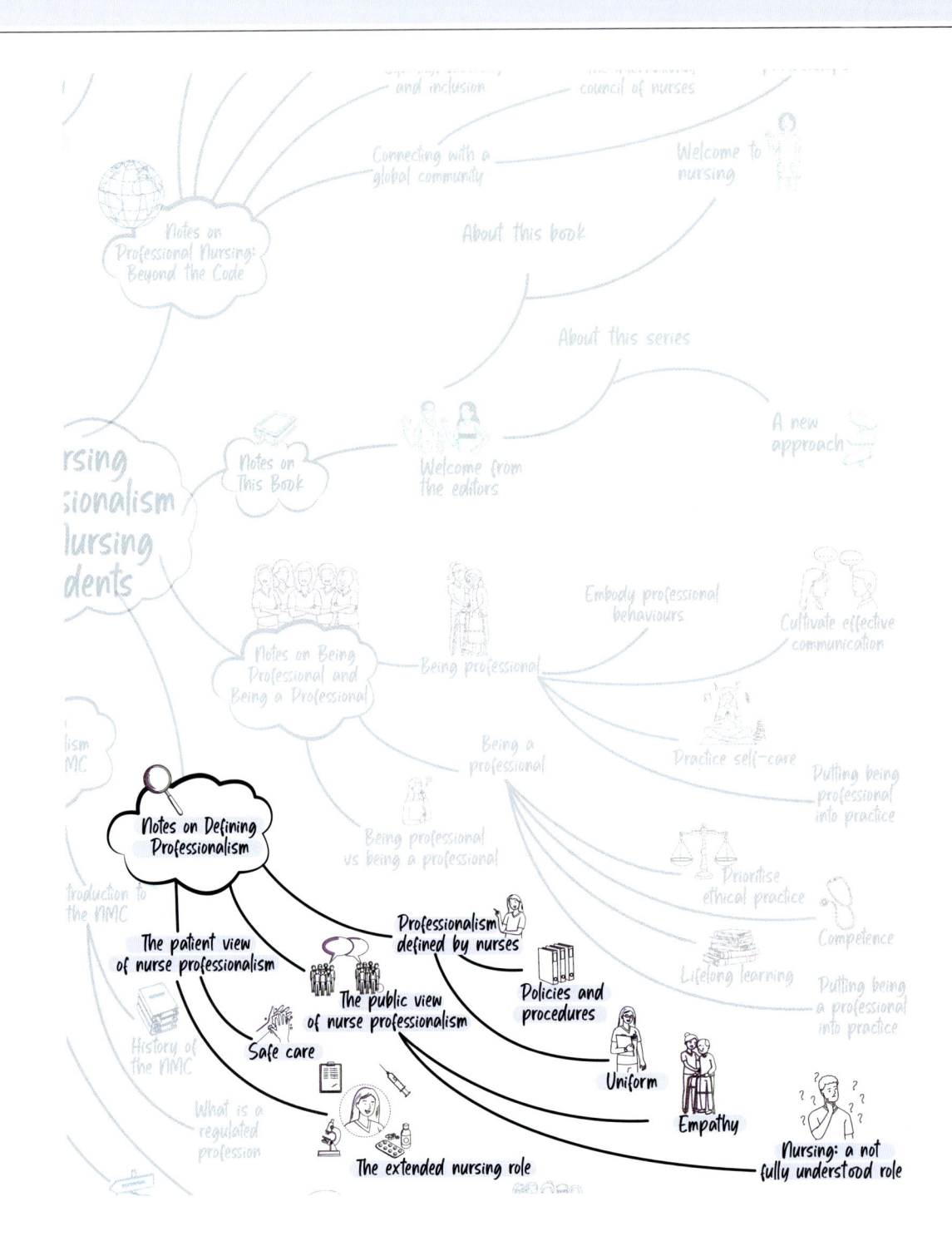

Notes on Defining Professionalism

- The patient view of nurse professionalism
- Professionalism defined by nurses
- The public view of nurse professionalism
- Safe care
- Policies and procedures
- Uniform
- Empathy
- The extended nursing role
- Nursing: a not fully understood role

NOTES ON DEFINING PROFESSIONALISM

Katharine Caddick (she/her)

INTRODUCTION

Nurses' identities are held in values and beliefs and guiding interactions with patients and professionals. The social image of nursing professionalism is part of that identity. Thoughts and professionalism are intertwined with the respect and deeply held values that nurses work towards. The guidance given by the 'code' from the Nursing and Midwifery Council (NMC) helps draw boundaries and clarify roles and responsibilities for us to uphold the respect of the profession as a whole. Ideas about professionalism reflect experiences throughout a nurse's career. Professionalism is not a solution or answer but rather a discussion that raises questions honestly and the sharing of personal experiences as a professional nurse and the identity and values that help. This chapter aims to explore all of this and, ultimately, how we define professionalism in nursing.

HOW DOES A NURSE BECOME A PROFESSIONAL?

Nursing and professionalism is, of course, not just about it being a job, qualification, role, or academic achievement. Neither is it simply what happens when we qualify. Professionalism is learned. There is a process of conforming to instruction, training and learning; a way to dress and speak to convey skill, competence and care; and having both distance and discipline while remaining warm and caring (Grinberg & Sela 2022).

> **SOCIAL MEDIA X**
> @punc22x
>
> Being professional means that one must uphold the NMC within and outside of work. It is also fundamental to treat every member of our global community with respect, dignity and care.

> **SOCIAL MEDIA X**
> @LaurenPUNC22
>
> Being a professional to me means acting in a way that's respectful to others and myself too. Acting with thought, maturity and consideration for my actions.

> **SOCIAL MEDIA X**
> @PUNC22NicMcMaho
>
> To me being a professional means being qualified, skilled, knowledgeable and competent in your specialised field of work whilst demonstrating the ability to behave in a conscientious, courteous and respectful manner.

Within nursing, females make up the most significant proportion of staff, and it's important to realise that, historically, females have struggled to be recognised and respected as professionals. Within nursing, the Regulation of Nurses Act was passed for England, Scotland, Wales and Ireland in 1919, meaning that all nurses had to learn the same subjects and meet the same standards, and they were recognised professionals (Royal College of Nursing 2017). This historical perspective still impacts nursing today, as nurses can still often feel like their autonomy is questioned or overlooked for those roles mistakenly assumed as more masculine, such as medicine (Lotan 2019, Grinberg and Sela 2022). Therefore becoming a professional in nursing can sometimes feel like an uphill struggle. There is absolutely no doubt that nursing professionals have autonomy and accountability. We have a huge responsibility and advocate care. We don't just fill gaps in the doctors' roles (even if, at times, we do). We don't just help doctors, (again, even if, at times, we do). But by no means is that the scope or breadth of any nurse. Rather, these are assets that are consistent and learned. Nursing is a highly skilled and distinct practice (Rodríguez-Pérez et al. 2022). Effective relationships and collaboration are required between doctors and nurses to achieve positive medical results (Mahboube et al. 2019), and this is something that nursing students need to develop and strengthen in their practice.

Professionalism and the code

The meaning of professionalism varies across time, cultures and contacts, and it's difficult to define (Cao et al. 2023). It's not just values or behaviours. It's a more complex concept of self-identity and characteristics that can be learnt and defined. All of this means that nursing professionalism plays a central role in clinical nursing. However, ultimately, professionalism is reaching a standard that is recognised and maintained, and professional values align with the code of conduct we adhere to. The NMC is clear that professionalism is not negotiable. The standards to be reached are absolute through all levels of experience. Nursing is bound up with the profession and development of the nursing role. We commit to professionalism when we become nurses. Anyone practising as a nurse in the United Kingdom or a nursing associate in England should have values and identities that match. The professional expectation of the NMC is to have a clear, consistent, positive message to nurse colleagues, teams, other healthcare professionals and society as a whole—about who we are and what we as nurses and society can expect.

> **SOCIAL MEDIA X**
> **@NMCnews**
>
> Our **Code** is clear that professionals should treat people fairly and challenge discrimination towards those receiving care, as well as when directed towards their colleagues.

> **SOCIAL MEDIA X**
> **@NMCnews**
>
> Our **Code** is clear that professionals on our register must promote professionalism and trust at all times. Where concerns are raised with us, we'll always look into it and consider taking action if needed.

> **SOCIAL MEDIA X**
> **@NMCnews**
>
> Treating people with kindness, compassion and respect is one of the first requirements of The **Code**. Thank you to the nurses, midwives & nursing associates on our register who uphold this value every day.

Nurses are expected to reinforce professionalism to obviously adhere to the rules and standards and provide ongoing evidence they are doing that. There must be continued learning, good practice and accepting of rules and authority. When exploring defining professionalism in nursing revalidation, the process by which all nurses need to follow to maintain their registration (NMC 2021) is part of that. Revalidation is not an option if we wish to continue practising as nurses.

2 | NOTES ON DEFINING PROFESSIONALISM

> **THE NMC SAYS**
>
> **6.2** Maintain the knowledge and skills you need for safe and effective practice.

Fig. 2.1 shows the revalidation requirements that nurses must meet every 3 years in order to be able to continue to practise.

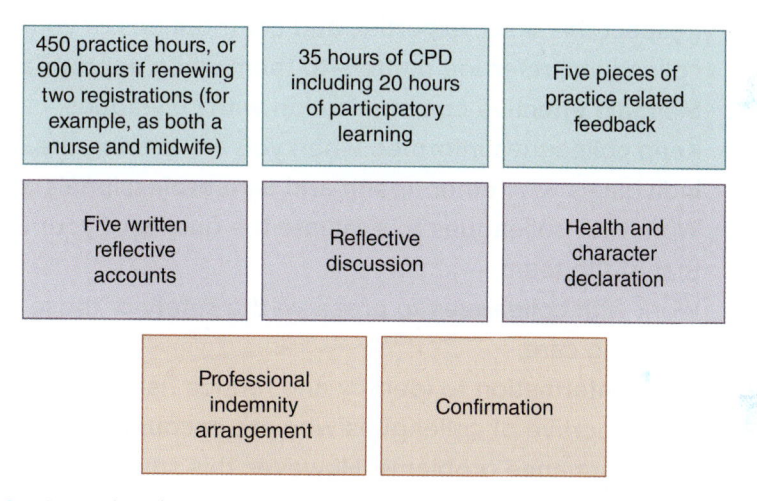

450 practice hours, or 900 hours if renewing two registrations (for example, as both a nurse and midwife)	35 hours of CPD including 20 hours of participatory learning	Five pieces of practice related feedback
Five written reflective accounts	Reflective discussion	Health and character declaration
Professional indemnity arrangement	Confirmation	

Figure 2.1 Revalidation requirements by nurses. *CPD*, Continuing professional development.

Revalidation is closely interwoven with the code and is therefore closely interwoven with defining professionalism in nursing.

> **SOCIAL MEDIA X**
> **@AndreaHarr15**
>
> Revalidation supports my practice and **professionalism** providing a framework. I reflect more since revalidation was introduced.

Defining professional relationships

Professionalism promotes safe collaboration, giving grounded and exacting levels of understanding of capability, education, trust and ability (Brennan and Monsoon 2014). The NMC Code talks at length about working with others and professional relationships.

THE NMC SAYS

8 Work cooperatively
   8.1 Respect the skills, expertise and contributions of your colleagues, referring matters to them when appropriate.
   8.2 Maintain effective communication with colleagues.
   8.3 Keep colleagues informed when you are sharing the care of individuals with other health and care professionals and staff.
   8.4 Work with colleagues to evaluate the quality of your work and that of the team.
   8.5 Work with colleagues to preserve the safety of those receiving care.
   8.6 Share information to identify and reduce risk.
   8.7 Be supportive of colleagues who are encountering health or performance problems. However, this support must never compromise or be at the expense of patient or public safety.
9 Share your skills, knowledge and experience for the benefit of people receiving care and your colleagues.
   9.1 Provide honest, accurate and constructive feedback to colleagues.
   9.2 Gather and reflect on feedback from a variety of sources, using it to improve your practice and performance.
   9.3 Deal with differences of professional opinion with colleagues by discussion and informed debate, respecting their views and opinions and behaving in a professional way at all times.
   9.4 Support students' and colleagues' learning to help them develop their professional competence and confidence.

2 | NOTES ON DEFINING PROFESSIONALISM

Professionalism should allow for discussion and cooperation between colleagues, discussing areas of concern without blame, looking for solutions and skills that can be shared. You can trust their experience, wisdom and expertise. Even junior nurses' professionalism can enhance standards amongst senior colleagues. We can learn from each other when we are confident of the standards.

> **SOCIAL MEDIA X**
> @MichelleSobande
>
> Remember that even the most experienced staff are still learning & often learn a lot by seeing things through the eye of students.

> **SOCIAL MEDIA X**
> @JaneMCummings
>
> Revalidation links our **professionalism** with our practice and our Code.

Lack of professionalism can lead to mistrust because there is no consistency or reliability. Development is unachievable, and relationships are damaged. It is important that practice should be challenged when professionalism is not seen to be achieved, and the NMC Code is clear on what to do if you have concerns.

> **THE NMC SAYS**
>
> **16** Act without delay if you believe that there is a risk to patient safety or public protection
> To achieve this, you must:
> **16.1** Raise and, if necessary, escalate any concerns you may have about patient or public safety, or the level of care people are receiving in your workplace or any other health and care setting and use the channels available to you in line with our guidance and your local working practices.

Continued

NMC

16.2 Raise your concerns immediately if you are being asked to practise beyond your role, experience and training.

16.3 Tell someone in authority at the first reasonable opportunity if you experience problems that may prevent you working within the Code or other national standards, taking prompt action to tackle the causes of concern if you can.

16.4 Acknowledge and act on all concerns raised to you, investigating, escalating or dealing with those concerns where it is appropriate for you to do so.

16.5 Not obstruct, intimidate, victimise or in any way hinder a colleague, member of staff, person you care for or member of the public who wants to raise a concern.

16.6 Protect anyone you have management responsibility for from any harm, detriment, victimisation or unwarranted treatment after a concern is raised.

17 Raise concerns immediately if you believe a person is vulnerable or at risk and needs extra support and protection
To achieve this, you must:

17.1 Take all reasonable steps to protect people who are vulnerable or at risk from harm, neglect or abuse.

17.2 Share information if you believe someone may be at risk of harm, in line with the laws relating to the disclosure of information.

17.3 Have knowledge of and keep to the relevant laws and policies about protecting and caring for vulnerable people.

There is equity in professionalism, a shared understanding, goals and values to promote people, work in partnerships, and respect, support, and provide compassion. There is an unspoken expectation that your colleagues are doing this too. There are no cut corners. Nurses do everything to 100%. When your colleagues' values and identity do not match the professionalism that nurses are called to, the distress and resentment it causes between staff and service users is evident. When you see something that is wrong, don't walk away—walk towards. Keep confidentiality and respect, dignity and kindness.

2 | NOTES ON DEFINING PROFESSIONALISM

> **CASE STUDY**
>
> Naomi is a registered nurse whose colleague failed to revalidate in time and was suspended while she waited for her pin to be reinstated. Naomi reflected on her thoughts and feelings around her colleague's actions:
>
> *The consequence of my colleague failing to revalidate left me feeling unsupported, upset and angry. She left me with not only my job but her job to do as well, so both our jobs are affected. I had to work hard to ensure that the trust that service users had in our care was maintained. My feelings towards my colleague became damaged as she didn't seem to think that it was her fault that the deadline was missed. She remains incredulous to the reaction of the NMC and the NHS Hospital Trust following their rules.*
>
> After a week, Naomi's colleague returned, and Naomi reflected again:
>
> *She's back now and I feel quite separated from her. Her clinical capability and level of education are not a question, but her professionalism is. She didn't fulfil her revalidation requirements, so how can I trust that she's in work or keeping her skills up to date? When one area of professionalism is not reached that causes the others to be questioned. This situation has shown me the impact of other people's unprofessional behaviour on the people we care for and the nursing team. As a registered nurse I have a responsibility to ensure that my registration remains up to date because the consequences of my registration lapsing are far reaching.*
>
> Naomi was placed under pressure due to her colleague's actions but was able to reflect on the importance of professionalism and her own responsibilities as a nurse.

Nurses should be accountable for their professionalism and practice and the care they give. That way, colleagues and other nurses can rely on them to achieve what is expected and accept responsibility (Cao et al. 2023). Professional standards and rules keep us in step together. It is important that there is a challenge to those who are not walking in step if their behaviour, attitude and values are not appropriately matched. If your colleague has not met the requirements, then we have all not met the requirements. Trust is lost by both the public and other nurses (Gallup 2022). We are accountable for our actions and inactions. We can't cover someone else's failings. However, when professionalism is reached, communication with colleagues is effective and informative, comprehensive and respectful. It supports and enhances performance to keep patients, colleagues and the public safe.

> **TIPS**
>
> Remember:
>
> - Your actions are about you—so know the standards, know the risks and work within the boundaries that keep people we care about safe.
> - If you have concerns about a colleague's professionalism, it is important that you raise them.
> - Write your concerns down so that you don't forget anything; try and stick to the facts.
> - Speak to someone more senior that you trust—this can be either at university or on placement.
> - Keep an accurate record of your actions.
> - Ensure that confidentiality is maintained.
> - Refer to your university and/or placement policy on whistleblowing.
> - Refer to the NMC, Raising Concerns Guidance for Nurses, Midwives and Nursing Associates (2019).

How will you ensure that your relationships with colleagues remain professional? Think about the professional qualities you have seen in nurses you know or encountered.

_____

_____

_____

_____

Professionalism as defined by nurses

Nurses feel passionately that being professional is about caring for people and showing empathy—not displaying care because we are being told to but rather because we identify with the values of the profession. It is a result of our professional identity, rather than managerial coercion. Nursing professionalism gives an importance to our work. It is identified with the successful and effective delivery of care, rather than targets that benefit a firm (Kenny et al. 2011, Mueller et al. 2008).

Nurses who understand what they signed up to be and how they respect and care, while being continually educated, are upholding the NMC values: prioritise people, practise effectively, preserve safety and promote professionalism and trust. Huber (2015) and Kenny et al. (2011) both talk about how following organisational policies and procedures and adhering to the rules of the governing body, organisation and educational body reduce risk and increase safety and confidence in what nurses are doing. But what do nurses themselves say? How do nurses define professionalism?

> **SOCIAL MEDIA X**
> **@Susan_Kent2**
>
> **Professionalism** requires us to be: knowledgeable, advocates, accountable, moral, ethical, innovative and entrepreneurial.

> **SOCIAL MEDIA X**
> **@KeelingJoanne**
>
> **Professionalism** doesn't mean nursing isn't fun. Some of the best times had are laughing with patients, carers and colleagues..good for the soul. We need to promote this aspect of our profession.

> **SOCIAL MEDIA X**
> **@MaryDunningTU**
>
> lifting the words off the paper, putting into practice. **Professionalism** involves the small things as well as the big things. The small things can have a big impact.

As nursing students, you will come across and work alongside many great nurses whose behaviours and actions encompass professionalism. They will inspire and support you over your career, and they will pull you and other colleagues into their standards simply by working in step with them.

> 'My first ward manager modelled her own professionalism. Sandra had insight and compassion. She was empathetic and available and held respect while being respectful. She was emotionally aware and honest. She demonstrated professionalism, advocacy, and accountability. She was able to guide me and step in gently where my role was not defined, to set professional expectations and to drive my standards forward. My identity reflected her understanding of professionalism. My education and training were not in doubt, we all started at the same level, but my ability to be a nurse was. By deliberately identifying with someone whose values were clearly aligned to the NMC and my own, I was able to observe what was required and develop my identity and professionalism'.
>
> *Anonymous, registered nurse*

> 'Peter was driven. Clear and precise. Full of knowledge and standards. He was inspiring. An expert. Professional. He strongly influenced my professional values of accountability and reliability. He was fully capable. He provided clarity and safe effective care through independent thought and vision. He was reliable and had the respected gravitas of experience and research. His professionalism was built on the expectations that he had of himself to fully embrace the NMC code. He had a clear history of working at a level of responsibility over a long time and was trusted to develop the service. He epitomised professionalism in work and mirroring the behaviour that is expected

2 | NOTES ON DEFINING PROFESSIONALISM

of a nurse outside work. He continued to strive for this, not only for himself, but for those around him and the service. He called out unprofessionalism and inadequacy. His professional identity as a nurse leader shaped the way he worked and interacted with others. He led the service with determination and inspiration. Peter was a brilliant professional and cared deeply. He was aware that there were other teammates who communicated more effectively than he did and so he delegated to make patient care constructive. Encouraging colleagues to step in where he had gaps. In this way, protecting the professionalism of the whole team. He recognised that it was his responsibility to engage successfully with other professionals for safe, effective care and the growth of the service to be productive'.

Anonymous, registered nurse

'Tracey was honest with integrity and empathy, coaching and developing staff for whom she had accountability. She was not clinical but, as a nurse manager, afforded space and direction to help her team develop the professional responsibility to work together and bring safe care. She learned to suspend her own judgements of people to support the nurse she was working with to reach their own understanding, professionalism and potential, whether this was within educational goals, revalidation, delivery of care. This developed my self-identity and lifted my own professionalism'.

Anonymous, registered nurse

Each nurse you work with will have their own view on professionalism and what it looks like; however, as shown in the testimonies, there are likely to be common themes, as outlined in Fig. 2.2.

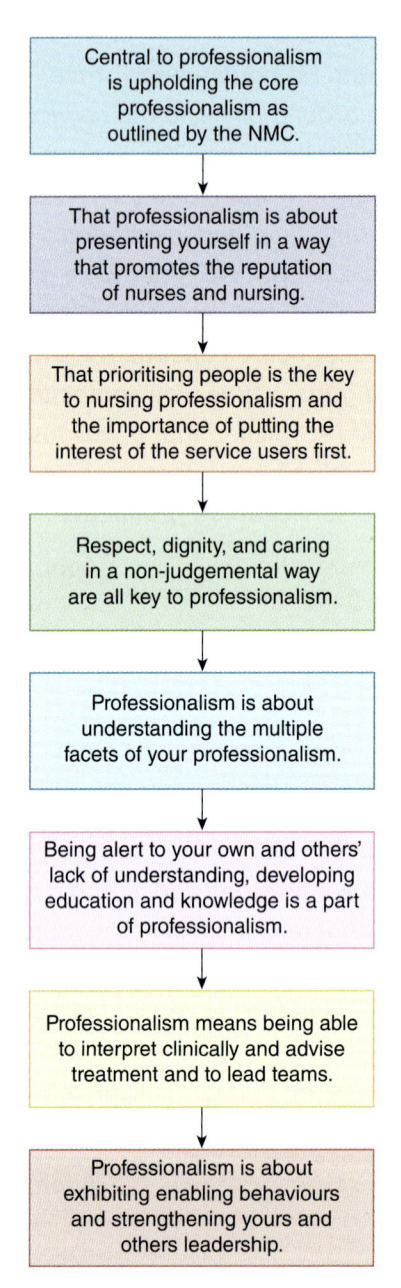

```
Central to professionalism
is upholding the core
professionalism as
outlined by the NMC.
        ↓
That professionalism is about
presenting yourself in a way
that promotes the reputation
of nurses and nursing.
        ↓
That prioritising people is the key
to nursing professionalism and
the importance of putting the
interest of the service users first.
        ↓
Respect, dignity, and caring
in a non-judgemental way
are all key to professionalism.
        ↓
Professionalism is about
understanding the multiple
facets of your professionalism.
        ↓
Being alert to your own and others'
lack of understanding, developing
education and knowledge is a part
of professionalism.
        ↓
Professionalism means being able
to interpret clinically and advise
treatment and to lead teams.
        ↓
Professionalism is about
exhibiting enabling behaviours
and strengthening yours and
others leadership.
```

Figure 2.2 Testimonies showing nurses' views on professionalism. *NMC*, Nursing and Midwifery Council.

2 | NOTES ON DEFINING PROFESSIONALISM

> **How do you define professionalism?**
>
> _____
> _____
> _____
> _____
> _____

The public view of professionalism in nursing

The role of a registered nurse is often misunderstood until people need one and see the breadth and scope of nursing for themselves. There is an understanding that we are highly educated and that it is often higher than public sector managers and business leaders. Does the public know that all registered nurses qualify with degrees? Or that senior nurses have master's degrees, with some achieving PhDs? That many nurses prescribe independently? Or work autonomously? It's safe to say that the public's view of nursing has not yet caught up with nurses being expert practitioners in their own right (Hoeve et al. 2014). The nursing horizon and achievements that scientific nursing can achieve, the advancing practice we strive for to fulfil our potential, is fast moving and constantly changing, so it is understandable that professionalism is not clearly defined for the public.

Nurses believe patients and the public remain unaware of what is involved in nursing professional performance. Indeed, even nursing students have a lack of knowledge of this. Some, even as they start with a degree, are not able to express what nursing was, or is (Mohamed 2013, Rodríguez-Pérez et al. 2022).

The following quote identifies the lack of understanding that the public has of nurses. Even someone who has known the nurse for a long time misunderstood the scope of their role and abilities.

> 'Recently a long-term friend was astonished that I teach doctors and have autonomy and can choose to remove stitches without the doctor telling me when.
>
> My elderly neighbour refers to her senior clinical nurse specialist and advanced practitioner as 'lovely girls', kind and helpful.
>
> This sentiment is commended, obviously, but she has little understanding of the deep knowledge and scientific research and the independent thinking and responsibility that her nurses hold.
>
> An elderly gentleman in my specialist clinic wanted to know my qualifications before I saw him; I doubt he would've asked a doctor that. I am confident that the doctors in my team would have deferred the answers to me as the expert in that field.
>
> Another patient having a procedure that I teach asked for the doctor I was teaching to do the procedure and not me because I was a nurse. I would've agreed, apart from the doctor I was teaching had never done this procedure. I do over 300 a year and teach the foundation doctors regionally as an expert. The patient's perception was that I was helping—filling in the gap—handing the doctor instruments'.
>
> **Anonymous, registered nurse**

Interestingly, studies show that patients have higher levels of trust in nurses and prefer them to convey emotionally difficult information over doctors (Girvin et al. 2016). The public's perception is that nurses will allow patients more time and are better equipped to give emotional care and support.

THE NMC SAYS

Promote professionalism and trust

You uphold the reputation of your profession at all times. You should display a personal commitment to the standards of practice and behaviour set out in the Code. You should be a model of integrity and leadership for others to aspire to. This should lead to trust and confidence in the profession from patients, people receiving care, other health and care professionals, and the public.

The public compares us to other healthcare professionals. The resulting explanation of what a nurse is and does is often mistaken and misrepresented. But nurses are autonomous, responsible for managing nursing care and are accountable for the appropriate delegation and supervision of care provided by others in the team, including the lay carer. They play an active and equal role in the interdisciplinary team, collaborating and communicating with a range of colleagues, working autonomously or as an equal partner with a range of other healthcare professionals and teams. Nurses provide leadership, coordinating compassionate, evidence-based and person-centred care. They are accountable for their own actions, not being told what to do by another healthcare professional.

Patients view professional competence in nursing as technical ability and knowledge (Calman 2006). There is an assumption that their care is safe. The patient knows that the nurse is registered and attributes competence and professionalism jointly to the grade of the nurse. There are clear competencies and standards that nurses need to reach to practise. These are to protect patients. The practice of nursing does not always fit the expectations of patients who, like the public, have a poor understanding of what a nurse does (Girvin et al. 2016, Thomas et al. 2019).

COVID AND POST–COVID PUBLIC PERCEPTION OF NURSING

Throughout the COVID pandemic, the public recognised, for the first time, that the identity of a nurse is in nursing itself and the desire to care and give to others, even in a crisis. Nurses were publicly visible in a way that they had never been before. Nurses were not just helping doctors or looking after hygiene; they had the answers and emotional resilience to help people. Public opinion changed about our ability and altruism. It was obvious that we were driven, passionate, resolute professionals all working together under frightening and overwhelming circumstances. Nurses were taking the lead in society as a way out of fear by keeping people safe and alive. Nurses were on the TV and radio. People saw nurses on the news—our hospitals being paralysed by the number of patients. Nurses and doctors were being honest, showing their fear and distress. The public recognised that in the signs of alarm throughout the world, nurses and all healthcare professionals remained focused, rational, organised, efficient and expert. Nurses were seen to be deliberately stepping into a situation that, in the minds of the country and world, was obviously frightening and dangerous (Tepperman 2020).

In the wake of COVID, the pressure on the NHS and healthcare has been highlighted. It is understood by the public that it is caused by a lack of provision and long-term lack of funding from the government (The Kings Fund 2019, NHS 2022). The public has since seen nurses campaigning for a pay raise to overcome years of real-term pay cuts and to protect patient safety.

'We strike for fairness. We strike for the future of our NHS. We strike because it's our right – and our duty – to stand up for fair pay and for patient safety. It is not unreasonable to demand better. This is not something that can wait. We are committed to our patients and always will be' (Cullen, 2022).

The public can see that all registered nurses who are part of the Royal College of Nursing—whether in the NHS or not—are standing together, upholding their professional standards and calling out failings and inadequacy that are damaging patient care.

The professionalism shown during strike action was underlined by the NMC, who updated their existing statement on industrial action by stressing that the 2023 NMC Code of Conduct still applies to nurses on the register while they are taking part in industrial action or are on strike. The standards of professional behaviours that the public has a right to expect from their nurses, midwives and nursing associates will continue to apply (NMC 2023).

The Observer Poll (Savage 2022) showed that the first strike, in December 2022, had high levels of support from the public. Over 60% of the public recognised that nurses were struggling, reporting that they supported the strike (Helm 2023). Pressure on the government from nursing unions was supported by the public as they identified with the frustrations of the NHS: the wearing down of public services, the pressure in the hospitals and the lack of communication between the nurses and the government. There was acknowledgement by the government that the nurses have public support more than other striking sectors, such as rail on the post office (Helm 2023).

Throughout the strikes, nurses were committed to continuing life-preserving services, including emergency intervention for the preservation of life or the prevention of permanent disability—and urgent diagnostic procedures and assessment required obtaining information on potentially life-threatening conditions or conditions that could potentially lead to permanent disability.

ENHANCING THE PUBLIC'S PERCEPTION

There is evidence of strong public trust, although this does not seem to be developed from an understanding of nurse work or impact (Girvin et al. 2016). It seems to be more from the respect of the traditional, sentimental and hard-working young females. Overall, the public is not clear about what a nurse does (Hayes 2019, Mohamed 2013, Sreeja and Nageshwar 2018). As a profession, we need to get better at promoting our skills and roles so that we are more visible. Society needs to be made aware of nurses; this can only be done by the nurses themselves. The public expects nurses' values to be related to personal, rather than professional, competence—a vocational study that doesn't quite match up with medicine. Professions with fewer males are considered 'female' and thus related less to power and more to caring (Rezaei-Adaryani et al. 2012). Nurses are seen as inferior to other healthcare professional team members and perceived as a secondary role to the doctors (Rodríguez-Pérez et al. 2022). This subordinate assumption influences the self-perception and identity of nurses themselves, making it difficult for nurses to display their professionalism and express their expertise (Sreeja and Nageshwar 2018).

The public perception of nurses as professionals can be enhanced by public awareness. The solution in the mismatch of projected and perceived images must come from the nurses themselves (Rodríguez-Pérez et al. 2022). Nurses need to take on leadership, teaching, political and high-level research roles. We need to highlight what we are doing by using traditional and social media, making nursing research more visible, and both nurses and nursing students have a role to play in doing this. To make a change in the perceived professional role, nurses need to identify as professional. We need to increase our self-esteem and rise up, train and encourage nursing students to proactively believe and display professionalism and equality with other healthcare professionals (Cao et al. 2023). Increased perceptions of nursing as a profession can be through raising societal awareness and also by enhancing the self-esteem of nurses. Nurses are the only ones who can make a change to the perceived image of nursing as a profession (Sreeja and Nageshwar 2018).

How will you enhance the public's perception of nursing?

The physical conditions, presentation of staff, as well as the attitude of colleagues and culture of the organization, all have a bearing on patients' perception of nurses' professionalism (Kenny et al. 2011). The demographic characteristics of patients, gender and culture will influence the patient's perceptions of what professionalism looks like in nursing (Cao et al. 2023). Can a young female nurse be professional? Does she need to be older to be in leadership, or should she be a male? What if she is wearing scrubs or a uniform dress? Does this alter how she is viewed? Nursing is perceived as a healthcare profession whose primary function is to care (Rodríguez-Pérez et al. 2022). It is assumed that males are typically managers, whereas females are typically caring (Rezaei-Adaryani 2012).

The interpersonal attributes and accessibility of the nurse, observed competence and feeling listened to, are all quality indicators in the patient's view of the nurse's professionalism (Thomas et al. 2019). The overarching view is that a nurse cares. It is reflected in the feeling that nursing is a vocation.

Patient and user involvement and empowerment are central to service development. Their views on nurses' professionalism and how competency is achieved are increasingly sought in healthcare (NHS Institute for Innovation and Improvement 2013). However, it is difficult to find an objective account of what patients feel about professionalism rather than how they feel cared for, even when they see nurses undertaking technical and unexpected roles.

Understanding the patient's experience is encouraged to match treatments to patient values and preferences (Knoepke 2022). Clearly, patients' opinions of nurses' professionalism are shaped by the length of time that they are cared for. This calls for consistency and recognition by the nurse that they are upholding their personal and professional reputation. The patient's perception of nursing will be affected in either a positive or negative way (Girvin et al. 2016, Knoepke 2022, Thomas et al. 2019).

It is unspoken but still assumed that nurses are being told what to do and when to employ our technical skills, rather than autonomously making decisions and sharing the responsibility with the healthcare team.

Of course, like everyone, a patient's personal views follow through their own worldviews and general attitudes. There are people throughout society who will uphold the view of the professional nurse, although some will assume that we are benefiting ourselves in some way, and they will never have a positive view of nurse professionalism.

> *'Patients often question why they're being told something by me—a senior nurse—even when I am clearly the expert. Patients look to the doctor for confirmation while the doctor is looking at me and relying on my knowledge.*
>
> *Conversely, other patients report that they could not have managed their treatments without my expertise, and that they would rather come to me to seek help to thank my medical colleagues as they recognise that I am the expert and am more accessible to them.*
>
> *I have been told by a patient that nurses make up rules for patients to help manage outcomes. Working within parameters that nurses set so that we care for people in a way that benefits us. He doesn't believe that we disclose the full information. He thinks we follow the mean of a curve and don't have to worry about personalised treatment plans. He believes that I am collecting data that benefits the hospital rather than the patient.*
>
> *Another patient reported that nurses that have looked after him in the past and coronary care have been helpful, but no more than that.*
>
> *Patients often comment that if my clinic is running behind, or that I arrive with a coffee that I haven't, that I am late, or haven't been doing anything. There is rarely the understanding that I have been called to see an urgent case, or I have a cold coffee that I've been holding all day long. In an increasingly immediate society, nurses are professional only when they deliver care that the patient expects on time as they want it.*
>
> *Others recognise and acknowledge that I am seeing extra patients and that I am stretching resources to give the best care'.*
>
> **Anonymous, registered nurse**

2 | NOTES ON DEFINING PROFESSIONALISM

Our professionalism must be in how we handle the mismatch between the perceived patient's view of the nursing role and what is actually happening (Girvin et al. 2016, Rodríguez-Pérez et al. 2022). Clearly, there are nurses who cut corners and don't demonstrate reassurance or communication. Thankfully, these are few, but again, they will be the ones that the patient will remember and will colour their opinion of all of us.

Importantly, it's recognised that patients trust information, diagnoses, prognoses and symptom control presented to them by a nurse (Gallup 2022, RCN 2022). Nurses report different roles in the processes of diagnostic and prognostic disclosures, including educator, care coordinator, supporter, facilitator and advocate (Newman 2016).

> What are your thoughts? Do we present information differently to doctors? Are we being viewed as less professional? Does that make us more approachable? Or is it that our role is to build trusting relationships with the patients in our care?
>
> _____
>
> _____
>
> _____
>
> _____

CONCLUSION

Nurses' professionalism is made up of a mixture of values and identity.

It is reliant on the nurse working within boundaries and their recognition of the guidelines presented by our governing body. It's also developed by the experiences that nurses encounter and their insight into the effect they have on peers, patients and the public.

It is important for nurses to develop self-awareness and consistency and to foster trust and professionalism in and out of work so that their care is reliable, regulated and effective.

Space for reader's own reflection:

REFERENCES

Brennan, D., Monsoon, V., 2014. Professionalism: Good for patients and Health Care Organisations. Mayo. Clin. Proc. 89 (5), 644–652.

Calman L., 2006. Patients' views of nurses' competence. Nurse. Educe. Pract. 6 (6), 411–417.

Cao, H., Song, Y., Wu, Y., Du, X., He, X., Chen, Y., et al., 2023. What is nursing professionalism? A concept analysis. BMC Nurs. 22 (1), 34. https://bmcnurs.biomedcentral.com/articles/10.1186/s12912-022-01161-0 [Accessed January 8, 2025]

Cullen, P., 2022. 'We strike for the future of the NHS': RCN strike action begins. Royal College of Nursing. https://www.rcn.org.uk/news-and-events/news/uk-rcn-nhs-nursing-strikes-2022-first-day-151222 [Accessed January 19, 2024]

Gallup. 2022. Honesty and Ethics in Professions. Gallup. https://news.gallup.com/poll/1654/honesty-ethics-professions.aspx [Accessed January 19, 2024]

Girvin, J., Jackson, D., Hutchinson, M., 2016. Contemporary public perceptions of nursing: A systematic review and narrative synthesis of the international research evidence. J. Nurs. Manag. 24 (8), 994–1006.

Grinberg, K., Sela, Y., 2022. Perception of the image of the nursing profession and its relationship with quality of care. BMC Nurs. 21, 57.

Hayes, C., 2019. 'As a society we need to reshape our perception of nursing.' Nursing Times. https://www.nursingtimes.net/students/as-a-society-we-need-to-reshape-our-perception-of-nursing-21-06-2019/#:~:text=However%2C%20I%20believe%20that%20as,challenging%20both%20emotionally%20and%20physically [Accessed January 19, 2024]

Hoeve, Y., Jansen, G., Roodbol, P., 2014. The nursing profession: Public image, self-concept and professional identity. J. Adv. Nurs. 70, 295–309.

Huber, T.H., 2015. Nursing professionalism. Ky. Nurse 63 (1), 15.

Knoepke, C.E., Chaussee, E.L., Matlock, D.D., 2022. Changes over Time in patient stated values and treatment preferences regarding aggressive therapies: Insights from the DECIDE-LVAD Trial. Med. Decis. Making 42 (3), 404–414.

Kenny, K., Whittle, A., Willmott, H., 2011. Understanding Identity and Organisations. Sage Publications Ltd, London.

Lotan, D.W., Taiar, R., 2019. Female nurses: Professional identity in question – how female nurses perceive their professional identity through their relationships with physicians. Cogent Med. 6 (1), 1648462. https://www.tandfonline.com/doi/full/10.1080/2331205X.2019.1648462 [Accessed January 8, 2025]

Mahboube, L., Talebi, E., Porouhan, P., Orak, R., Farahani, M., 2019. Comparing the attitude of doctors and nurses toward factors of collaborative relationships. J. Fam. Med. Prim. Care 8 (10), 3267–3272. https://doi.org/10.4103/jfmpc.jfmpc_644_19 [Accessed January 8, 2025]

Mohamed, L.K., 2013. Junior undergraduates nurse students' images of nursing as a career choice. Am. J. Sci. 9 (12), 25–34.

Mueller, F., Valsecchi, R., Smith, C., Gabe, J., Elston, M.A., 2008. 'We are nurses, we are supposed to care for people': Professional values among nurses in NHS Direct call centres. New Technol. Work. Employ. 23 (1–2), 2–17.

Newman, A., 2016. Nurses' perceptions of diagnosis and prognosis-related communication an integrative review. Cancer Nurs. 39 (5), 48–60.

NHS Institute for Innovation and Improvement. 2013. The Patient Experience Book. https://www.england.nhs.uk/improvement-hub/wp-content/uploads/sites/44/2017/11/Patient-Experience-Guidance-and-Support.pdf [Accessed January 19, 2024]

NMC. 2019. Raising concerns: Guidance for nurses, midwives and nursing associates. https://www.nmc.org.uk [Accessed January 3, 2025]

NMC. 2021. What is revalidation? https://www.nmc.org.uk/revalidation/overview/what-is-revalidation/ [Accessed January 18, 2024]

NHS. 2022. The NHS Long Term Plan: Overview and summary. https://www.longtermplan.nhs.uk/online-version/overview-and-summary/ [Accessed January 19, 2024]

NMC. 2023. Our position on industrial action. https://www.nmc.org.uk/news/news-and-updates/our-position-on-industrial-action/#:~:text=Nursing%20and%20midwifery%20professionals%20have,action%20or%20are%20on%20strike [Accessed January 18, 2024]

RCN. (2022). Nursing is the most trusted profession – it's official! [online]. https://www.rcn.org.uk/news-and-events/news/uk-nursing-most-trusted-profession-290322 [Accessed January 8, 2025]

Royal College of Nursing. 2022. Nursing confirmed as 'most trusted profession' as strike risk grows. https://www.rcn.org.uk/news-and-events/news/uk-nursing-confirmed-as-most-trusted-profession-as-strike-risk-grows-231122 [Accessed January 18, 2024]

Rezaei-Adaryani, M., Salsali, M., Mohammadi, E., 2012. Nursing image: An evolutionary concept analysis. Contemp. Nurse 43 (1), 82–90.

Rodríguez-Pérez, M., Mena-Navarro, F., Domínguez-Pichardo, A., Teresa-Morales, C., 2022. Current social perception of and value attached to nursing professionals' competences: An integrative review. Int. J. Environ. Res. Public Health 19 (3), 1817.

Royal College of Nursing. 2017. The Voice of Nursing. https://drive.google.com/drive/my-drive [Accessed January 19, 2024]

Savage, M., 2022. Public support for nurses' strike piles pressure on Sunak and divides Tories. The Guardian. https://www.theguardian.com/uk-news/2022/dec/17/public-support-nurses-strike-pressure-sunak-tories [Accessed January 19, 2024]

Sreeja, D., Nageshwar, V., 2018. Public perception of nursing as a profession. Int. J. Res. Appl. Sci. Biotechnol. 5 (5), 15–19. https://www.academia.edu/38972458/Public_Perception_of_Nursing_as_a_Profession [Accessed January 8, 2025]

Tepperman, J., 2020. Why Are We So Scared of the Coronavirus? FP. https://foreignpolicy.com/2020/03/11/coronavirus-global-panic/ [Accessed January 19, 2024]

The KingsFund. 2019. The NHS long-term plan explained. https://www.kingsfund.org.uk/publications/nhs-long-term-plan-explained [Accessed January 19, 2024]

Helm, T., 2023. Most UK voters still back strikes by nurses and ambulance crews. The Guardian. https://www.theguardian.com/politics/2023/jan/14/most-uk-voters-still-back-strikes-by-nurses-and-ambulance-crews [Accessed January 19, 2024]

Thomas, D., Newcomb, P., Fusco, P., 2019. Perception of caring among patients and nurses. J. Patient Exp. 6 (3), 194–200.

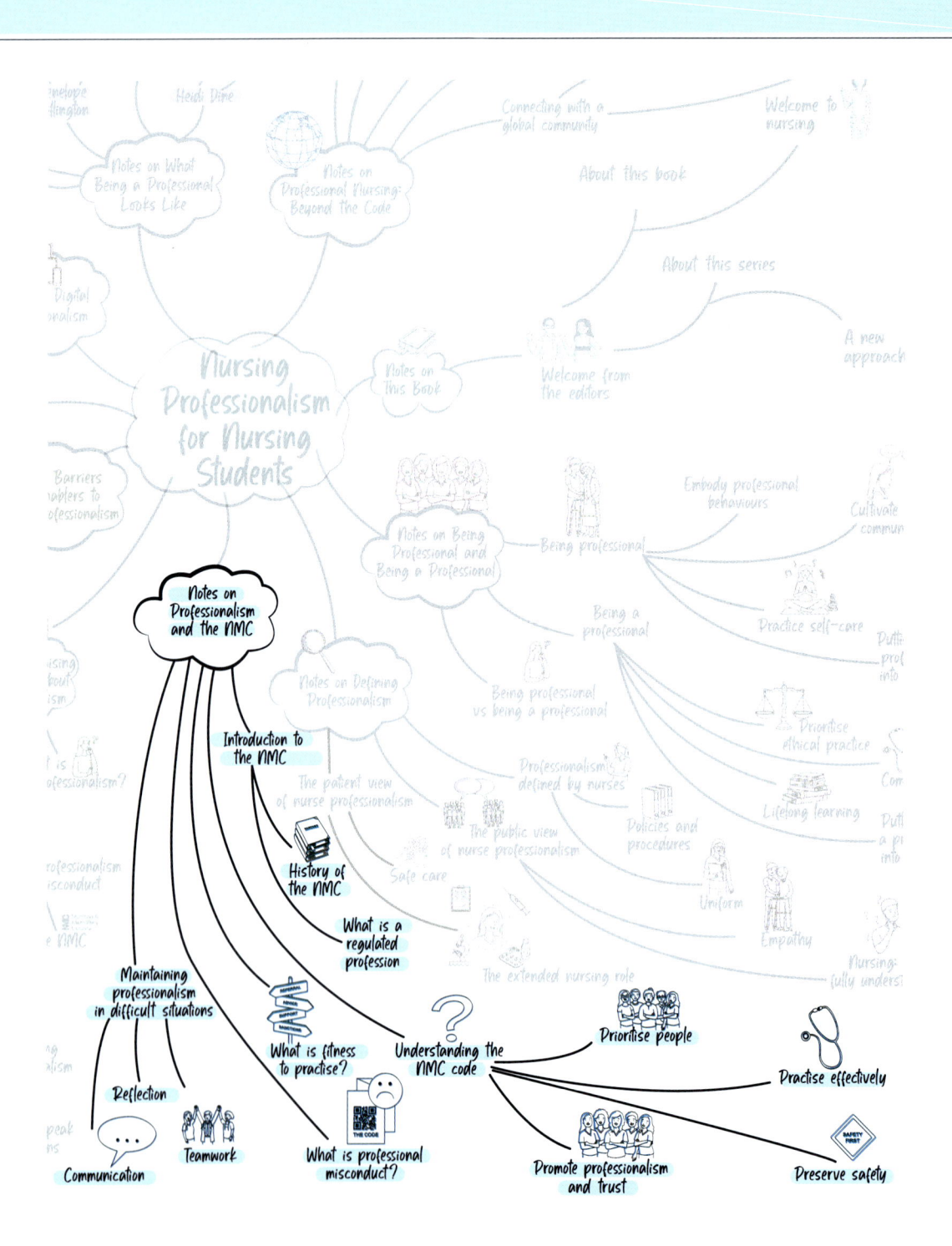

Notes on Professionalism and the NMC

- Introduction to the NMC
- History of the NMC
- What is a regulated profession
- Maintaining professionalism in difficult situations
  - Reflection
  - Communication
  - Teamwork
- What is fitness to practise?
- What is professional misconduct?
- Understanding the NMC code
  - Prioritise people
  - Practise effectively
  - Preserve safety
  - Promote professionalism and trust

NOTES ON PROFESSIONALISM AND THE NMC

Liz Grogan (she/her)

INTRODUCTION

This chapter introduces the reader to the regulatory body for nurses, midwives and nursing associates in the United Kingdom. It takes the reader through the areas such as fitness to practise, professional misconduct and maintaining professionalism in difficult situations. This chapter will use scenarios based on the cultural context of nursing as well as published fitness to practise cases from the Nursing and Midwifery Council (NMC).

The chapter will have four distinct sections:

- Introduction to the regulatory body
- Understanding the NMC code
- What is fitness to practise?
- What is professional misconduct?
- How do I maintain professionalism in difficult situations?

INTRODUCTION TO THE REGULATORY BODY

The history of the NMC

The NMC is the independent regulator for nurses and midwives in the United Kingdom and nursing associates in England.

> **NMC**
>
> **THE NMC SAYS**
>
> About us: The Nursing and Midwifery Council exists to protect the public. We do this by making sure that only those who meet our requirements are allowed to practise as a nurse or midwife in the UK, or a nursing associate in England. We take action if concerns are raised about whether a nurse, midwife or nursing associate is fit to practise.

Prior to 1919, there was no regulatory body for nurses in the United Kingdom. Ethel Gordon Fenwick, who was a matron at St Bartholomew's Hospital in London, spent 32 years campaigning for the registration of nurses. Ethel wanted to establish a mandatory register of nurses. In addition to this, she also wanted to standardise training, improve patient safety and advance the profession (Nursing and Midwifery Council 2019).

The NMC was first established as the General Nursing Council in 1919 as a regulatory body for nurses in the United Kingdom. The NMC (2019) stated that Ethel Gordon Fenwick 'watched from the public gallery in the House of Commons as the Nurses Registration Act was passed'. In 1923, Ethel became the first nurse registered in the United Kingdom—she was issued with badge number one (Nursing and Midwifery Council 2019)!

Fast forward to 1983, and the General Nursing Council was replaced with The United Kingdom Central Council for Nursing, Midwifery and Health Visiting, which, in 2002, became the NMC (Glasper and Carpenter 2019).

What is a regulated profession?

A regulated profession is a profession which is regulated by law in, or a part of, the United Kingdom. Regulators carry out a range of functions in relation to the professionals they regulate, including making sure people have the correct qualifications and experience to practise the profession and take the necessary enforcement action. A wide range of healthcare professionals are regulated, including doctors, dentists, radiographers, pharmacists, optometrists, speech and language therapists and many more (Gov.uk 2024).

The role of the NMC is to set standards for education, training and practise for nurses, midwives and nursing associates in the United Kingdom. The NMC plays a key role in ensuring the highest standards of care and professionalism are maintained in these vital healthcare professions.

The NMC is the regulatory body for nurses in the United Kingdom, where it operates across the four nations: England, Wales, Scotland and Northern Ireland. While the NMC establishes the standards and regulations applicable to all nurses, midwives and nursing associates, there are subtle differences in the application and oversight of these standards within each country.

The NMC sets standards for education, training and professional conduct to ensure that nurses meet professional standards and maintain their competence. The NMC supports students right from the start, telling students what they need to learn. The NMC sets standards on what nursing students should be taught so that when a student qualifies, they can step into their first job with the right skills and knowledge to care for people safely and effectively.

The NMC keeps a register so that employers can check who can work as a nurse, midwife or nursing associate—there are currently more than 690,000 people on the NMC register. The NMC expects all of these registered nurses, midwives and nursing associates to work by the correct standards and uphold the code of practise throughout their entire careers. To ensure that people adhere to these standards every 3 years, each nurse, midwife and nursing associate must go through the process of revalidation. Revalidation shows the NMC that people are continuing to learn and develop and reflect on their practise. Fig. 3.1 outlines the NMC's revalidation requirements that nurses, midwives and nursing associates must meet every 3 years; the NMC code is central to the revalidation process and can be used as the basis for professional reflection. Through revalidation, nurses provide rich evidence to demonstrate their ability to practise safely and effectively (Ashurst 2017).

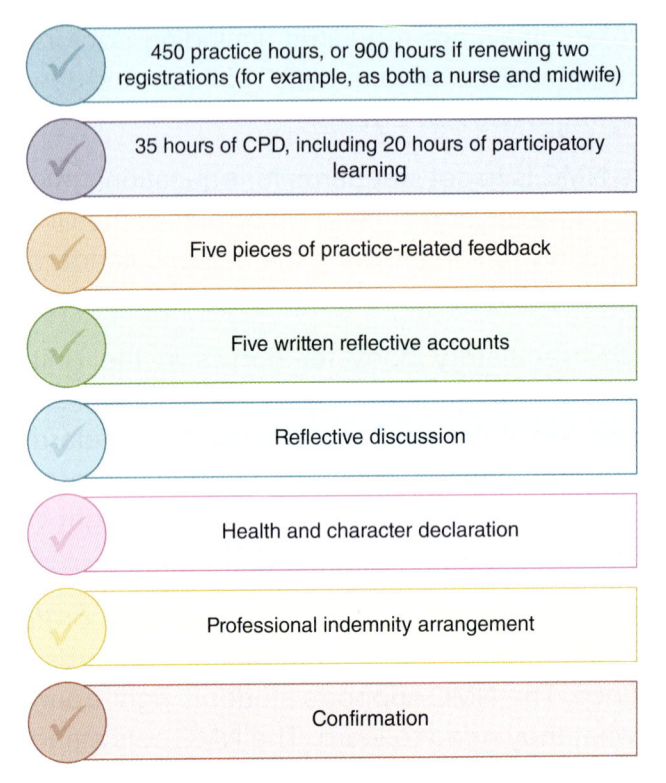

- 450 practice hours, or 900 hours if renewing two registrations (for example, as both a nurse and midwife)
- 35 hours of CPD, including 20 hours of participatory learning
- Five pieces of practice-related feedback
- Five written reflective accounts
- Reflective discussion
- Health and character declaration
- Professional indemnity arrangement
- Confirmation

Figure 3.1   NMC revalidation requirements.

UNDERSTANDING THE NMC CODE

The NMC code presents the professional standards that nurses, midwives and nursing associates must uphold in order to be registered to practise in the United Kingdom (England only for nursing associates). The code sets out common standards of conduct and behaviour for those on our register. This provides a clear, consistent and positive message to patients, service users and colleagues about what they can expect of those who provide nursing or midwifery care.

> **THE NMC SAYS**
>
> **20** Uphold the reputation of your profession at all times.

3 | NOTES ON PROFESSIONALISM AND THE NMC

The NMC code is structured around four themes:

- prioritise people
- practise effectively
- preserve safety
- promote professionalism and trust

Each section contains a series of statements that, taken together, signify what good nursing and midwifery practise look like.

What does prioritising people mean?

- Put the interests of people using or needing nursing or midwifery services first.
- Make sure their care is your main concern.
- Make sure that their dignity is preserved.
- Their needs are recognised, assessed and responded to.
- People are treated with respect, and their rights are upheld.
- Any discriminatory attitudes and behaviours are challenged.

> *'From nursing on the ward followed by being an orthopaedic sister and then the lead practice development nurse, prioritising people has always been at the centre of everything and every evidenced-based decision I have made in my nursing career. It doesn't matter which nursing job you do; you will always be prioritising people. This has driven me as a nurse to ensure I am providing the best care; whether it is hands-on care or via education and teaching staff who are delivering the care to patients.*
>
> *When I was nursing on an orthopaedic ward, I would be prioritising people depending on their health and holistic needs. Patients are most vulnerable when they are in hospital or a care setting and we are their advocate; it is important to build a professional relationship with your patients. My priority would always be a critically ill patient or a deteriorating patient who needs urgent medical care. However, the holistic side of nursing is equally important. I have spent many hours*

Continued

on each shift talking to patients about their lives, their families, pets and what is important to them to ensure they feel safe, as it is an unfamiliar and sometimes frightening time for patients being in hospital'.

Hannah Welbourne, RN, MSc, PGCert, clinical placement lead

What does practise effectively mean?

- Deliver and assess needs of your patient or advise on treatment or give help without too much delay to the best of your abilities.
- Practice is in line with the best available evidence.
- Communicate clearly, with accurate records and sharing skills.
- Reflect and act on feedback to improve your practice.

'Practising effectively means to me that the nurse has:

- *Knowledge and understanding of the Nursing Midwifery Council Code of Conduct. The nurse adheres to expected standards, including maintaining confidentiality, advocating for patients and treating all with respect.*
- *Clear and effective communication skills. To be able to convey and receive information.*
- *The right level of knowledge, skills, attitude and ability, to be clinically competent to deliver safe and effective person-centred care.*
- *The ability to build a trustworthy and professional relationship with those in their care and those they work with.*
- *Clinical judgement, critical thinking and problem-solving skills and can use them effectively when assessing, planning, delivering and evaluating care.*
- *The motivation and commitment to continue with their lifelong learning. Keeping up to date with current and new trends, along with embracing technological advancements to enhance patient care.*

3 | NOTES ON PROFESSIONALISM AND THE NMC

> - *The aptitude to work both independently and within a team. They are willing to share their knowledge and skills, as well as being receptive to learning from others.*
> - *Clear understanding of the term's accountability and responsibility in relation to their role and when delegating duties to others'.*
>
> **Heather Short, MSc, BSc, DipDn, RGN**

How would you preserve safety?

- Make sure that patient and public safety is not compromised.
- Work within your limits of competence, exercising professional 'duty of candour', and raise concerns immediately of situations that may put patients or public safety at risk.
- Take appropriate action to deal with any concerns where necessary.

> 『 *'Preserving safety is one of the four standards expected of nurses, nursing associates and midwives, as outlined in the Nursing and Midwifery Council Code.*
>
> *Nurses, nursing associates and midwives work within a multitude of settings and frequently need to make complex decisions, often as part of a multiprofessional team.*
>
> *As registrants of the Nursing and Midwifery Council in the United Kingdom, we are reminded that we must make sure that patient and public safety is not affected by our actions. We are encouraged to work within the limits of our competence, exercising our professional 'duty of candour' and raising concerns whenever we come across situations that put patients or public safety at risk. Irrespective of seniority and/or experience, we are all required to take necessary action to deal with any concerns where appropriate.*
>
> *The Code contains a series of statements that, taken together, signify what good practice by nurses, midwives and nursing associates looks*

Continued

> *like. It puts the interests of patients and service users first, is safe and effective, and promotes trust through professionalism'.*
>
> **Steve Hams, Chief Nursing Officer, North Bristol NHS Trust**

How would you promote professionalism and trust?

- You would, at all times, uphold the reputation of the profession.
- Demonstrate and display a personal commitment to the standards of practise.
- Be a role model of integrity and leadership for others to aspire to.
- This should lead to patients, healthcare professionals and the public having trust and confidence in you.

> *'Promoting professionalism and trust as a nurse might sound complex. I believe, however, this is at the heart of what being a nurse truly means. Building trust with the people around you, whether they are patients, service users, relatives or colleagues, means communicating well and building successful relationships. Ultimately, this allows you to advocate for those who need it most. Nurses are skilled, knowledgeable professionals who also get to be right at the bedside (or clinic/telephone!) of someone who needs care. I think being professional in the role is not just about following specific policies (although of course, that is very important!) but also about how you act on a daily basis. This means keeping up to date with your clinical knowledge, being accountable for your actions and upholding a high standard of care, and you should be able to expect the same from your colleagues. Being a nurse also means you are in an important position of acting as a role model to others, including student nurses and experienced nurses who are new to the NMC register. Supporting each other to adhere to these standards encourages a good culture and ultimately improves patient care'.*
>
> **Zoe Hill, RN, clinical education lead**

> ✏️ What are your thoughts on the NMC code? How will you ensure that you take all four themes into account in your daily practise?
>
> _____
> _____
> _____
> _____
> _____
> _____

What is the duty of candour?

Candour means being honest and telling the truth, especially in relation to difficult subjects (Cambridge Dictionary n.d.) The NMC is clear about nurses, midwives and nursing associates' duty of candour:

> **THE NMC SAYS**
>
> Preserve safety: You make sure that patient and public safety is not affected. You work within the limits of your competence, exercising your professional "duty of candour" and raising concerns immediately whenever you come across situations that put patients or public safety at risk. You take necessary action to deal with any concerns where appropriate.

Griffith et al. (2019) explains that 'imposing a professional duty of candour on all registered health professionals, and this includes nurses, ensures a consistent approach to candour and the reporting of errors. A professional duty also ensures that those who seek to obstruct others in raising concerns will be in breach of their professional code and guilty of professional misconduct'.

> What qualities as a nurse do you think you need to maintain a duty of candour? (Some keywords might be: open and honest, be prepared to apologise, effective communication, embrace learning culture.)
>
> _____
> _____
> _____
> _____
> _____
> _____

The standards expected of nurses

According to Griffith et al. (2019), professionalism can be defined as the competence, skills and values expected of a registered nurse, midwife or nursing associate, and this is a key theme of the NMC code—emphasising the need to promote professionalism and trust. The NMC's role is to set the standards in the code, but it is important to remember that these aren't just the NMC's standards; they are the standards that the patient and members of the public expect from healthcare professionals. They are the standards shown every day by those on the NMC register.

The NMC provides a clear framework through the code of practise for registrants to follow in terms of their professional and ethical obligations, emphasising how this promotes consistency and fairness across the profession. In addition, nurses, midwives and nursing associates are expected to work within the limits of their competence, which may extend beyond the standards they demonstrated in order to join the register.

3 | NOTES ON PROFESSIONALISM AND THE NMC

> **TIPS**
> Remember, it's okay to say no! If there is a clinical skill that you feel you are not competent in delivering, it's important that you say so. As nurses, it's okay to say no and then address the gap in knowledge or skills and seek to learn more and become competent. If you do not feel competent in catheterising a patient or undertaking an aseptic technique procedure, it's important to say no, and do not put the patient at risk of unsafe practise.

WHAT IS FITNESS TO PRACTISE?

Sometimes things can go wrong, and people might have concerns about a nurse, midwife or nursing associate; the NMC can investigate these concerns and take action where needed to protect patients. The NMC's fitness to practise process investigates complaints and takes disciplinary action against nurses who breach its code of ethics and standards. This process can result in outcomes such as suspension or removal from the nursing register.

The NMC works with employers and healthcare organisations to prevent issues that may lead to fitness to practise hearings and provides support to nurses going through the process.

The NMC ensures fairness and impartiality during fitness to practise hearings and communicates the outcomes to the public and stakeholders. The NMC's regulatory framework promotes professionalism, ethical conduct and ongoing learning and development in nursing practise. However, events such as the Letby trial question the credibility of nurses and the trust that the general public has in the profession.

> **CASE STUDY**
> **Letby trial**
> This case relates to a high-profile murder enquiry where the nurse was criminally charged with seven counts of murder and seven counts of attempted murder (against six victims) involving neonatal babies. The nurse put patients, as a consequence of their own actions, at unwarranted risk of harm. There was clear evidence that harm was repeated and deliberate. Letby abused her position of trust as a nursing professional, demonstrated a pattern of offending over an extended period of time and has, to date, shown no remorse for her actions, evidencing attitudinal issues. The individual breached all aspects of the code. The panel considered a number of passages from the judge's sentencing, including:
>
> *'You acted in a way that was completely contrary to the normal human instincts of nurturing and caring for babies and in gross breach of the trust that all citizens place in those who work in the medical and caring professions. The babies you harmed were born prematurely and some were at risk of not surviving, but in each case you deliberately harmed them intending to kill them'* (Nursing and Midwifery Council 2023a).
>
> The sanction imposed by the panel, after careful consideration, was a striking-off order—the individual has been struck off the register.

Fitness to practise is about keeping people safe as opposed to punishing people on the register. Our roles are set out in the code, and for a nurse, midwife or nursing associate, the NMC must make sure that their skills, knowledge, education or behaviour do not fall below these standards needed to deliver safe, effective and kind care. Fitness to practise cases like the Letby case are in the minority; however, the case did distress many nurses and nursing students. The Chief Nursing Officer of England, Dame Ruth May (2023), stated, 'Colleagues within the nursing profession and across the health service have been shocked and sickened to learn what she did, actions beyond belief to the nurses and staff working so hard to save lives and care for patients'.

> How do you feel when there is a large number of articles in the press about trials such as the Letby case?
>
> _____
> _____
> _____
> _____
> _____
> _____

Concerns raised and investigated by the NMC about nurses, midwives and nursing associates are something that affect a tiny minority of professionals each year. The fitness to practise process allows the NMC to understand as quickly as possible whether a registered professional presents a risk to the public. If they do, steps can be taken to promote learning and prevent issues from arising again. However, to put fitness to practise into context, during the period between 2022 and 2023, there were a total of 3348 new referrals made to the NMC out of over 690,000 people on the NMC register (Health and Care Professions Council 2022). Fig. 3.2 shows some reasons why nurses, midwives and nursing associates have been referred to the NMC for fitness to practise:

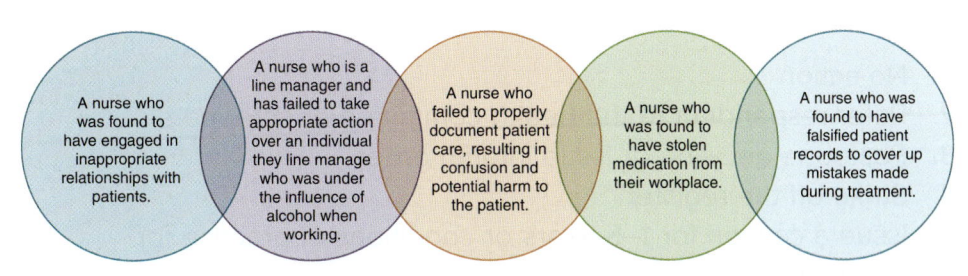

- A nurse who was found to have engaged in inappropriate relationships with patients.
- A nurse who is a line manager and has failed to take appropriate action over an individual they line manage who was under the influence of alcohol when working.
- A nurse who failed to properly document patient care, resulting in confusion and potential harm to the patient.
- A nurse who was found to have stolen medication from their workplace.
- A nurse who was found to have falsified patient records to cover up mistakes made during treatment.

Figure 3.2 NMC fitness to practice referral reasons.

> **TIPS**
> Fitness to practise hearings are held in public so nursing students can arrange to watch a hearing. This is a good way to really understand the fitness to practise process. Contact the NMC to arrange shadowing of a fitness to practise hearing, either virtually or face to face.

For most nurses and midwives, the thought of being referred to their regulator is a very scary thing. According to Hathaway (2017), 'Many do not engage, finding the whole process too stressful and intimidating from the outset, and imagining only one outcome: striking off'.

> **TIPS**
> Being a member of a union, such as the Royal College of Nursing (RCN) or UNISON, is a good way to ensure that if you ever need legal representation at a fitness to practise hearing, you have it. A union can support you through any investigations or any complaints, worries or concerns you have.

What powers does a fitness to practise committee have?

Following an investigation and referral to a fitness to practise committee, after a finding of unfitness to practise, the committee can take one of the following actions:

1. No action
2. Refer respondent to the health committee or screeners
3. Postpone decision or issue interim order
4. Strike off the register
5. Issue a caution for 1–5 years or conditions of practise for 1–3 years
6. Suspend from register for up to 1 year

The case studies that follow are examples of fitness to practise cases.

CASE STUDY

Failures around clinical care (Nursing and Midwifery Council 2023b):

This case is about a nurse who was reported to the NMC following an allegation against them for falsifying records. The alleged falsified records suggested that the nurse undertook a home visit to a patient. There were questions raised over the records being inaccurate because of the condition of the patient's bandages were found in and the patient's claim of not being visited. This was taken to a fitness to practise panel, and evidence was received from a witness called on behalf of the NMC that called the nurse's practise into question. The NMC had a legal assessor as part of the panel and referred to guidance relating to the specific charges. The NMC report references the full deliberation and charges raised against the nurse. The ultimate sanction was that the nurse was suspended for a period of 12 months with a review.

CASE STUDY

Racial discrimination (Nursing and Midwifery Council 2024):

This case relates to an individual who was referred by their employer to the NMC for allegations of racial discrimination and referring to colleagues in a derogatory way with the use of deeply offensive racist words. A number of charges were laid out against the individual. The report highlights that 'registered nurses occupy a position of privilege and trust in society and are expected at all times to be professional and to maintain professional boundaries. Patients and their families must be able to trust nurses with their lives and the lives of their loved ones'. The panel deemed that there had been a serious breach of the code, as the individual failed to uphold the standards and values of the nursing profession, therefore bringing the reputation of the profession into disrepute. As a consequence, the sanction for the individual was an interim suspension of 18 months; if no appeal was made, then the individual would receive a striking-off order.

CASE STUDY

Sexual harassment (Nursing and Midwifery Council 2023c):

This case relates to a nurse who was referred to the NMC for breaching professional boundaries and breaching of confidentiality by accessing private information about a colleague. The panel found a number of the charges were proven, and due to limited circumstantial evidence, others were not proven. The panel then considered the nurse's fitness to practice, and as a result of the misconduct, the individual's fitness to practise was deemed impaired. The panel considered the judgement of Mrs. Justice Cox in the case of CHRE v NMC and Grant in reaching its decision:

'In determining whether a practitioner's fitness to practise is impaired by reason of misconduct, the relevant panel should generally consider not only whether the practitioner continues to present a risk to members of the public in his or her current role, but also whether the need to uphold proper professional standards and public confidence in the profession would be undermined if a finding of impairment were not made in the particular circumstances'.

The sanction imposed over the individual was a caution order over a 3-year period.

What are your thoughts on the fitness to practise case studies?

_____
_____
_____
_____
_____
_____

What are the health consequences of fitness to practise cases?

According to Dean (2017), 'Of the complaints about a specific profession in hospital and community care, 26% related to nurses'. Concerns can be raised from employers, patients/members of the public and colleagues. The NMC clearly states that the best way to deal with internal complaints made in NHS trusts is through local investigation and resolution as long as it does not leave the public at risk. Fitness to practise will always remain a vital part of the NMC's function and is paramount to ensuring patient safety. In many cases, the registrant is striving for the best for their patients, keeping them at the centre of what they do.

> 'I have a had a few really positive few week's feeling much better and sleeping uninterrupted, but then I received a letter in the post and I have a pending hearing, I was referred 7 months ago—I just feel so anxious and worried all the time—I love my job'.
>
> **Molly, registered nurse**

In 2018–19, the NMC's annual report (Glasper and Carpenter 2019) highlighted that four nurses were recorded as having died by suicide while undergoing fitness to practise investigations. The fitness to practise process can do severe harm to nurses, who go through long-term psychological effects from the process. Even if there is 'no case to answer', registrants can feel lost, let down and lacking in confidence, and some have reported elements of posttraumatic stress disorder (Dean 2020).

> **TIPS**
>
> All of the outcomes of fitness to practise cases are on the NMC website; in order to get to grips with professionalism and the role the NMC plays, it is a good idea to read through some of the most recent cases. Simply search 'Latest hearings and sanctions' on the NMC website.

What support can I get if referred to the NMC?

- Nurses have access to a free emotional support service established by the NMC in 2019. The confidential 24-hour service is operated by an independent provider.
- Registrants can access structured counselling sessions, delivered either face to face, via phone or video call, or online using email or a secure chat room.
- The Samaritans offer a safe place to talk any time, including about job-related stress or anxiety. Call free on 116 123.
- The RCN can put its members in touch with their other services that can offer help, including immigration, employment legal advice and financial support. Contact the fitness to practise care line by calling 0800 587 7396.
- There is a fitness to practise library which is also a helpful resource; search 'Fitness to practise library' on the NMC website (Foster 2024).

WHAT IS PROFESSIONAL MISCONDUCT?

Nurses, midwives and nursing associates play a vital role in ensuring patients' well-being and recovery. They are patients' trustworthy caregivers, advocates and instructors (Audrey et al. 2021). Professional misconduct refers to any practice or action by nurses that deviates from the established ethical and professional standards and guidelines (Currie et al. 2019, Hulme et al. 2019). Essentially, professional misconduct is where a registrant has failed to meet and violated the standards outlined in the code.

More than 170,000 complaints were made in England about patient care during 2021 and 2022—and the actual figure of complaints may be higher due to challenges recording data during COVID-19 (Dean 2017). Evidence suggests that the main themes for complaints are communication, patient care and staff values and behaviours. Examples of conduct that could lead to conduct and competence proceeding are outlined in Fig. 3.3 (unprofessional behaviours in the workplace—a level of incivility), which can be described as being rude or discourteous or having disrespectful actions, can also be constituted as professional misconduct.

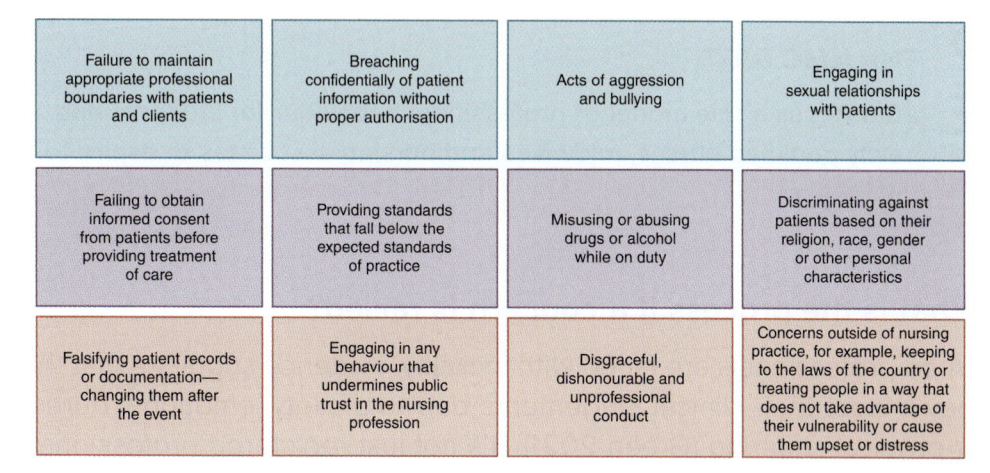

Failure to maintain appropriate professional boundaries with patients and clients	Breaching confidentially of patient information without proper authorisation	Acts of aggression and bullying	Engaging in sexual relationships with patients
Failing to obtain informed consent from patients before providing treatment of care	Providing standards that fall below the expected standards of practice	Misusing or abusing drugs or alcohol while on duty	Discriminating against patients based on their religion, race, gender or other personal characteristics
Falsifying patient records or documentation—changing them after the event	Engaging in any behaviour that undermines public trust in the nursing profession	Disgraceful, dishonourable and unprofessional conduct	Concerns outside of nursing practice, for example, keeping to the laws of the country or treating people in a way that does not take advantage of their vulnerability or cause them upset or distress

Figure 3.3 Examples of conduct that could lead to conduct and competence proceeding.

> ### THE NMC SAYS
>
> **Promote professionalism and trust**
>
> You uphold the reputation of your profession at all times. You should display a personal commitment to the standards of practise and behaviour set out in the Code. You should be a model of integrity and leadership for others to aspire to. This should lead to trust and confidence in the profession from patients, people receiving care, other health and care professionals and the public.

> ### THE NMC SAYS
>
> **20** Uphold the reputation of your profession at all times.
>
> To achieve this, you must:
>
> **20.1** Keep to and uphold the standards and values set out in the Code.
>
> **20.2** Act with honesty and integrity at all times, treating people fairly and without discrimination, bullying or harassment.
>
> **20.3** Be aware at all times of how your behaviour can affect and influence the behaviour of other people.

> **THE NMC SAYS**
>
> 20.8 Act as a role model of professional behaviour for students and newly qualified nurses, midwives and nursing associates to aspire to.

What is the process if a concern is raised?

When professionals are faced with incivility, evidence suggests that this may impact their clinical judgements due to anxiety, emotional duress or physical suffering (Green 2021). It's not just registered professionals who may experience this; nursing students have also reported experiences of bullying while on clinical placement (Birks et al. 2017, Houck and Colbert 2017). It is important that professional misconduct is reported. If a registrant's conduct falls short of the requirements of the code, what they did or failed to do could be severe enough for the NMC to take action.

What is important to remember is that not all breaches of the code or issues raised will be a matter of concern for the regulating body, and the NMC clearly states that many instances of misconduct are better dealt with by the employer in the first instance. Even when there has been significant and serious harm to people receiving care as a result of clinical error, provided there is no longer a risk to those receiving care and the registrant can demonstrate learning, the NMC usually does not need to take any further action.

HOW TO MAINTAIN PROFESSIONALISM IN DIFFICULT SITUATIONS

It's important to maintain a calm and respectful demeanour when faced with sensitive or confrontational situations. As healthcare professionals, we need to adhere to ethical and legal standards, even in the face of difficult circumstances or when under pressure, as outlined in the code.

3 | NOTES ON PROFESSIONALISM AND THE NMC

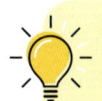

> **TIPS**
>
> Ali (2018) suggests the following tips for managing difficult situations:
> - 'Recognise that it is human to have feelings and emotions
> - Do not lose your temper; raise your voice; get angry, sarcastic or provocative; or attempt to humiliate the aggressor
> - Take a deep breath, relax, and remain calm, neutral and respectful
> - Do not react and start disagreeing: pause and think before acting
> - Say "no" to unreasonable demands, but be prepared to manage any adverse reaction
> - Do not tell the person that you know how they feel but do try to see the situation from their perspective
> - Show warmth and empathy
> - Do not let a bad experience with one person affect your whole day/shift or your family life—keep a sense of perspective and a professional attitude'.

Intrinsic factors also have a role in maintaining professionalism in difficult circumstances. Recognising that you may be tired or stressed on a shift that is short staffed will always result in challenging circumstances where professionalism is tested. Being able to appreciate that these things not only affects your own behaviour but also has an impact on others is a key nursing skill.

> **CASE STUDY**
>
> Beata is a third-year nursing student who is on placement on a busy surgical ward. Beata arrives on shift one day; it is her third day on duty, and she is feeling quite tired. Unfortunately, there are very few staff members on duty. Beata is allocated to work with her practise assessor for the day; however, almost immediately, her practise assessor gets called away to support another junior staff member with an emergency. Beata finds herself feeling stressed and overwhelmed. There are numerous call bells going off and lots of things on her to-do list. Another nurse asks Beata to help with something, and Beata snaps back that she doesn't have time.

Continued

> **CASE STUDY—cont'd**
>
> The nurse takes Beata to one side and takes an understanding approach, asking Beata if she is okay. Beata explains that she is feeling tired and stressed. The nurse listens and advises Beata to take 5 minutes to breathe and reflect. Beata steps away for 5 minutes and, with the help of the nurse, reflects on the shift and creates a plan for the morning. Beata finds that this really helps, and by the time her practise assessor returns, Beata is much less stressed.

Communication is key when dealing with difficult situations. It's important to be transparent, open and honest in all interactions with patients and colleagues and take the appropriate steps to address any mistakes or errors that may have occurred.

> **THE NMC SAYS**
>
> Preserve safety. You make sure that patient and public safety is not affected. You work within the limits of your competence, exercising your professional "duty of candour" and raising concerns immediately whenever you come across situations that put patients or public safety at risk. You take necessary action to deal with any concerns where appropriate.

Difficult situations can be de-escalated by employing communication strategies. Ali (2018) argues that 'good communication is often one of the first things to be abandoned in a challenging situation. We tend to stop listening to people we find challenging; our interruption rate increases; our body language can become closed and even hostile; we may be defensive; or become argumentative or difficult ourselves'. Some good ways to de-escalate a situation are presented in Fig. 3.4.

As nurses and nursing students, we all face difficult situations, and one of the most important things to do when faced with a difficult situation where your professionalism is tested is to learn and grow from it. Reflection and reflective practice play a really important part in professionalism in difficult

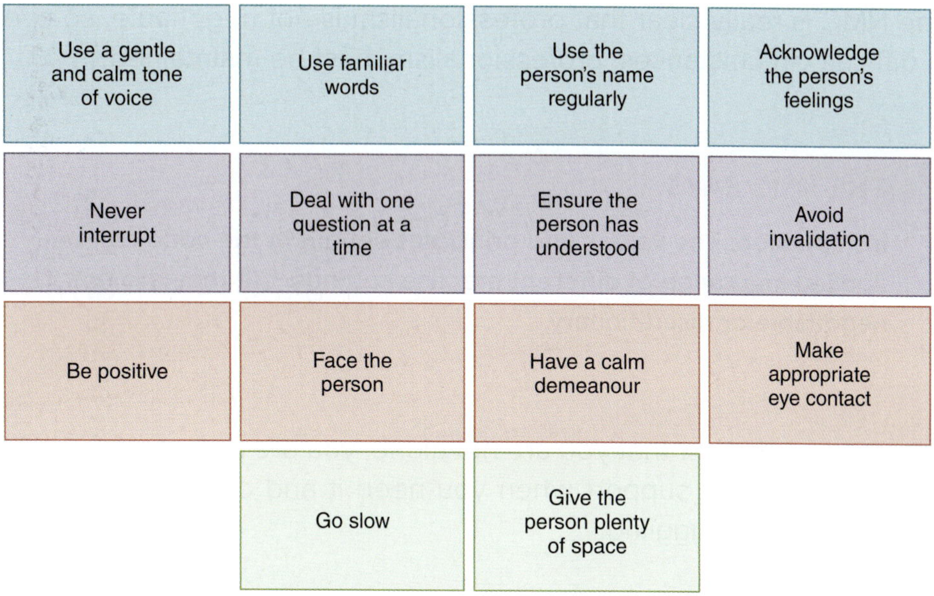

3 | NOTES ON PROFESSIONALISM AND THE NMC

Use a gentle and calm tone of voice	Use familiar words	Use the person's name regularly	Acknowledge the person's feelings
Never interrupt	Deal with one question at a time	Ensure the person has understood	Avoid invalidation
Be positive	Face the person	Have a calm demeanour	Make appropriate eye contact
	Go slow	Give the person plenty of space	

Figure 3.4 How to de-escalate a situation. (Adapted from Doncatser and Bassetlaw Teach Hospitals (2023) De-escalation: Principles and Guidance including Restraint [online] Available at: https://www.dbth.nhs.uk/wp-content/uploads/2023/07/De-escalation-Policy-PAT-PS-15v6.docx (Accessed: 11 April 2024).)

circumstances. Once the situation has died down, take time to think about what happened, what you did well and what you could have done better.

> Take 5 minutes to think about a difficult situation that you have had recently (it could be nursing related or personal). What did you do well? What could you have done better? Think about the NMC code while reflecting, and be really honest with yourself.
>
> _____
> _____
> _____
> _____
> _____

The NMC is really clear that professionalism is not negotiable, so even in difficult circumstances, professionalism must be maintained.

> **THE NMC SAYS**
>
> Introduction: The values and principles set out in the code can be applied in a range of different practise settings, but they are not negotiable or discretionary.

However, remember that you are not alone; you are part of a team. Use your team, ask for support when you need it and offer support when you see others struggling.

> **TIPS**
>
> A good way to help yourself or a colleague to maintain professionalism in a difficult situation is to take a break. Sometimes this feels counterintuitive, especially if there is a lot going on; however, even a short amount of time spent stepping away can provide a much-needed rest and time to reflect and regroup.

CONCLUSION

The NMC and the NMC code are integral to nursing professionalism. The NMC exists to protect the public, and this is done by clearly stating the values and principles that nurses, midwives and nursing associates should abide by.

The NMC is also responsible for investigations into professionalism in practise through fitness to practise. Although fitness to practise is a scary prospect for nurses, midwives and nursing associates and some examples shared in this chapter are very serious, it's important to remember that fitness to practise affects a minority of nurses, midwives and nursing associates.

The NMC can also take action in cases of professional misconduct, but this is not always the case, as many incidences of professional misconduct are dealt with by the employer in the first instance.

Maintaining professionalism in difficult situations is a challenge for all nurses, midwives and nursing associates, including nursing students. It is vital, though, for nursing students to understand that the NMC is clear that professionalism and the NMC code are not negotiable.

Ultimately, the NMC and nursing professionalism are intrinsically linked. Understanding how the NMC and the NMC code work, how fitness to practise and professionalism play a part and how to apply all of this in challenging circumstances are all key concepts to understand as a nursing student.

Space for reader's own reflection:

REFERENCES

Ali, M., 2018. Communication skills 6: Difficult and challenging conversations. Nurs. Times 114 (4), 51–53.

Ashurst, A., 2017. Understanding the Nursing and Midwifery Council's Code. Nurs. Resid. Care 19(5), 294–295.

Audrey, T., Berman, S.S., Frandsen, G., 2021. Kozier & Erb's Fundamentals of Nursing. Vol. 11. Pearson.

Birks, M., Cant, R.P., Budden, L.M., Russell-Westhead, M., Özçetin,Y.S.Ü., Tee, S., 2017. Uncovering degrees of workplace bullying: A comparison of baccalaureate nursing students' experiences during clinical placement in Australia and the UK. Nurse. Educ. Pract 25.

Cambridge Dictionary. n.d. Candour [online]. https://dictionary.cambridge.org/dictionary/english/candour [Accessed April 11, 2024]

Currie, G., Richmond, J., Faulconbridge, J., Gabbioneta, C., Muzio, D., 2019. Professional misconduct in healthcare: Setting out a research agenda for work sociology. Work. Employ. Soc 33(1), 149–161.

Dean, E., 2017. Professionalism. Emerg. Nurse 25(3), 13.

Dean, E., 2020. All you need to know about NMC fitness to practise case. Nurs. Stand 35 (8), 30–33.

Doncatser and Bassetlaw Teach Hospitals. 2023. De-escalation: Principles and Guidance including Restraint [online]. https://www.dbth.nhs.uk/wp-content/uploads/2023/07/De-escalation-Policy-PAT-PS-15v6.docx [Accessed April 11, 2024]

Foster, S., 2024. Fitness to Practise: The latest guidance. Br. J. Nurs 33 (6), 317.

Glasper, A., Carpenter, D., 2019. Celebrating 100 years of nurse regulation. Br. J. Nurs. 28 (22), 1490–1491.

Green, C., 2021. The hollow: A theory on workplace bullying in nursing practice. Nurs. Forum 56, 123–130.

Griffith, R.A., Dimond, B., Dowie, I., 2019. Dimond's Legal Aspects of Nursing. Pearson, UK.

Gov.uk. 2024. Professions regulated by law in the UK and their regulators [Online]. https://www.gov.uk/government/publications/professions-regulated-by-law-in-the-uk-and-their-regulators/uk-regulated-professions-and-their-regulators [Accessed April 11, 2024]

Hathaway, J., 2017. What midwives need to know about NMC Fitness to Practise hearings. Br. J. Midwifery 25 (4), 215–220.

Health and Care Professions Council. 2022. Whistleblowing Disclosures Report 2022 [Online]. https://www.hcpc-uk.org/globalassets/resources/2022/whistleblowing-disclosures-report-2022.pdf?v=637998773180000000 [Accessed April 11, 2024]

Houck, N.M., Colbert, A.M., 2017. Patient safety and workplace bullying: An integrative review. J. Nurs. Care. Qual. 32 (2), 164–171.

Hulme, S., Hughes, C.E., Nielsen, S., 2019. What factors contributed to the misconduct of health practitioners? An analysis of Australian cases involving the diversion and supply of pharmaceutical drugs for non-medical use between 2010 and 2016. Drug. Alcohol. Rev 38 (4), 366–376.

May, R., 2023. NHS England. Commenting on the verdict in the Lucy Letby trial [Online]. https://www.england.nhs.uk/2023/08/commenting-on-the-verdict-in-the-lucy-letby-trial/ [Accessed April 11, 2024]

Nursing and Midwifery Council. 2019. Always caring, always nursing [Online]. https://www.nmc.org.uk/news/press-releases/always-caring-always-nursing/ [Accessed April 11, 2024]

Nursing and Midwifery Council. 2023. Our role [Online]. https://www.nmc.org.uk/about-us/our-role/ [Accessed April 11, 2024]

Nursing and Midwifery Council. 2023a. Reasons: Fitness to practice C/SH-67757-20231212 [Online]. https://www.nmc.org.uk/globalassets/sitedocuments/fitness to practiceoutcomes/2023/december-2023/reasons-letby-fitness to practicecsh-67757-20231212.pdf [Accessed April 11, 2024]

Nursing and Midwifery Council. 2023b. Reasons: Fitness to practice C/SH-81777-20231124 [Online]. https://www.nmc.org.uk/globalassets/sitedocuments/fitness to practiceoutcomes/2023/november-2023/reasons-nkabinde-ftpcsh-81777-20231124.pdf [Accessed April 11, 2024]

Nursing and Midwifery Council. 2023c. Reasons: Fitness to practice C/SH-90573-20231120 [Online]. https://www.nmc.org.uk/globalassets/sitedocuments/fitness to practiceoutcomes/2023/november-2023/reasons-kyeremeh-ftpcsh-90573-20231120.pdf [Accessed April 11, 2024]

Nursing and Midwifery Council. 2024. Reasons: Fitness to practice C/SH-85144-20240105 [Online]. https://www.nmc.org.uk/globalassets/sitedocuments/fitness to practiceoutcomes/2024/january-2024/reasons-lesniak-ftpcsh-85144-20240105.pdf [Accessed April 11, 2024]

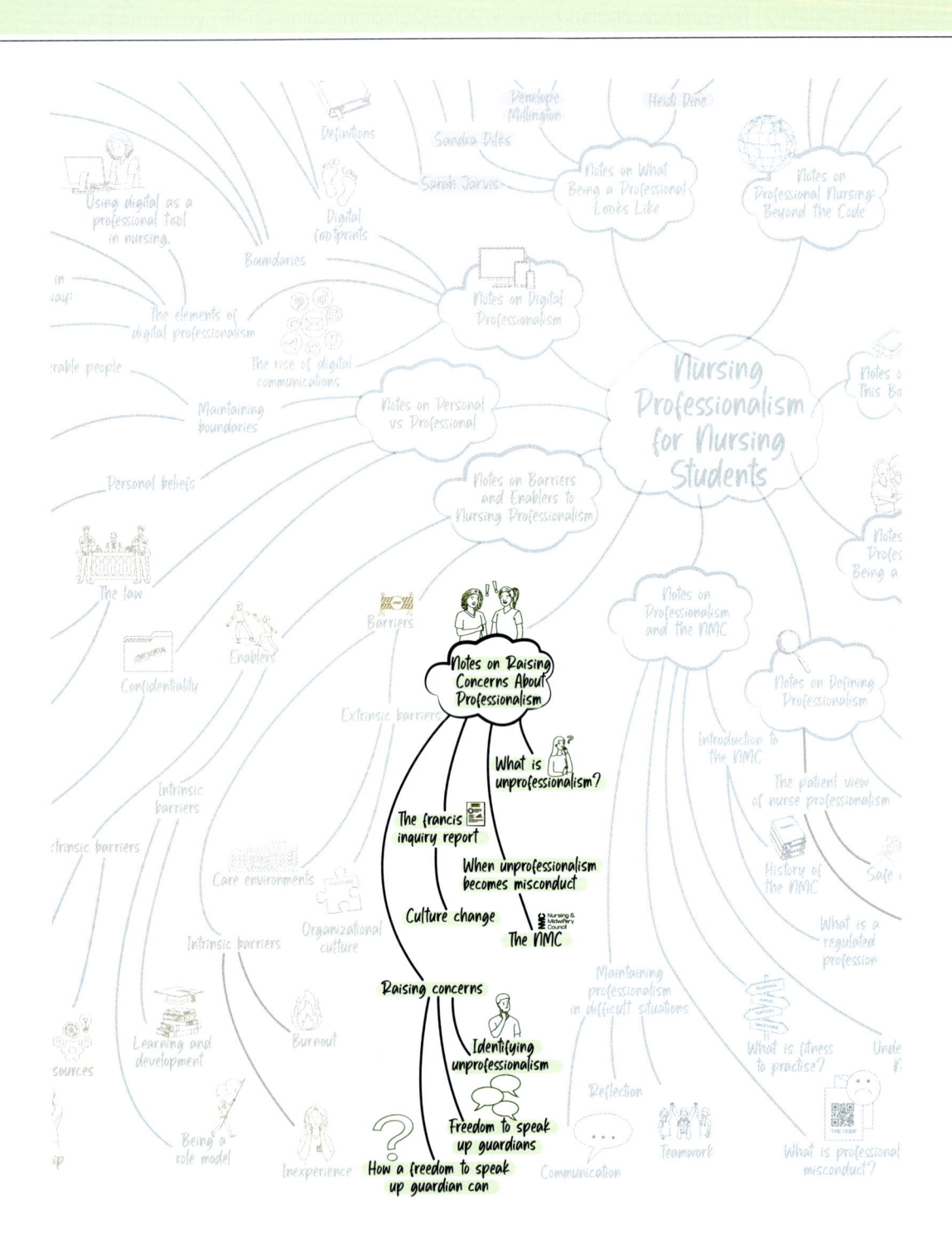

Nursing Professionalism for Nursing Students

Notes on Raising Concerns About Professionalism

- What is unprofessionalism?
- The Francis inquiry report
- When unprofessionalism becomes misconduct
- Culture change
- The NMC
- Raising concerns
- Identifying unprofessionalism
- Freedom to speak up guardians
- How a freedom to speak up guardian can

4

NOTES ON RAISING CONCERNS IDENTIFYING UNPROFESSIONALISM AND MAINTAINING SAFETY

■ Michelle Samson (she/her)   ■ Philip Ball (he/him)
■ Debra Hazeldine   ■ Teresa Chinn (she/her)

INTRODUCTION

Nurses, nursing associates and student nurses all have a professional responsibility to raise a concern (Nursing and Midwifery Council [NMC] code of conduct). All organisations will have processes available to use; this includes safeguarding processes/policies. Any team members raising any concerns will be supported by colleagues and a mentor. If it is felt that concerns are not being heard or dealt with, a concern can also be raised with the NMC or the Care Quality Commission (CQC).

> **THE NMC SAYS**
>
> **14** Be open and candid with all service users about all aspects of care and treatment, including when any mistakes or harm have taken place.

Continued

NMC

To achieve this, you must:

14.1 Act immediately to put right the situation if someone has suffered actual harm for any reason or an incident has happened which had the potential for harm.

14.2 Explain fully and promptly what has happened, including the likely effects, and apologise to the person affected and, where appropriate, their advocate, family, or carers.

14.3 Document all these events formally and take further action (escalate) if appropriate so they can be dealt with quickly.

16 Act without delay if you believe that there is a risk to patient safety or public protection.

To achieve this, you must:

16.1 Raise and, if necessary, escalate any concerns you may have about patient or public safety, or the level of care people are receiving in your workplace or any other health and care setting and use the channels available to you in line with our guidance and your local working practices.

16.2 Raise your concerns immediately if you are being asked to practise beyond your role, experience and training.

16.3 Tell someone in authority at the first reasonable opportunity if you experience problems that may prevent you working within the Code or other national standards, taking prompt action to tackle the causes of concern if you can.

16.4 Acknowledge and act on all concerns raised to you, investigating, escalating or dealing with those concerns where it is appropriate for you to do so.

16.5 Not obstruct, intimidate, victimise or in any way hinder a colleague, member of staff, person you care for or member of the public who wants to raise a concern.

16.6 Protect anyone you have management responsibility for from any harm, detriment, victimisation or unwarranted treatment after a concern is raised.

This chapter will explore the concept of not being professional and how to raise concerns if you feel, as a nursing student or once you have become a registered nurse, that safety and care have been compromised.

4 | NOTES ON RAISING CONCERNS IDENTIFYING UNPROFESSIONALISM

This chapter tells us much about being professional and ways in which being professional can be expressed, such as the NMC code of conduct. There are also examples in the quotes, each ultimately addressing the question: 'How do we raise concerns if we think a colleague is being unprofessional?'

WHY DOES PROFESSIONALISM MATTER?

This all ultimately matters, as professionalism helps us to deliver kind, caring and effective care. The following X (formerly Twitter) post from a patient highlights how important professionalism is:

> **SOCIAL MEDIA X**
> **@MarkyOatcake**
>
> On women's day here are some of the women that have shown such professionalism, nursing care & empathetic support over the past three years. I honestly don't know where I'd be today without their knowledge, skills & experience.

The impact that you may have on other people's lives may not always be explicitly known, but it can be quite profound. Sometimes the impact you have may not be immediate, or something that you view to be quite small could end up having a very big impact on someone else.

> **CASE STUDY**
>
> Shilpa is a nursing student who is working in a hospital ward setting where a patient in custody is admitted and allocated as one of her patients. This patient has three prison officers with them, and they are handcuffed to an officer at all times. Shilpa becomes aware that the patient has been involved in a high-profile offence where they have harmed children. Shilpa talks to her practice assessor and explains how she feels very uneasy about caring for this person, as she finds herself thinking about the victims of this person's crime.

Continued

CASE STUDY—cont'd

However, this patient has a wound that requires dressing. Shilpa asks her practice assessor how she maintains her professionalism while balancing her own morals and values. The practice assessor explains how she 'puts on her professional hat', and this helps her to remain emotionally competent, impartial and compassionate and remain an advocate for the people she cares for. The practice assessor points Shilpa to the NMC's 'Enabling Professionalism' document (NMC 2018) that outlines what professionalism looks like in practice, and she spends some time with Shilpa, role modelling how to balance personal feelings and professional actions. The practice assessor explains how debriefing and reflective discussions and writing can help with this balance and resilience in future situations like this.

Take some time to reflect on areas where your professionalism may be tested, like Shilpa's in the case study. Consider situations that you may find difficult and think about how you would manage this in practice. You may have already been in a situation where your professionalism was tested, and if so, consider how you dealt with this situation, and if you were in this situation again, would you do anything differently, and why?

Tips for how to maintain professionalism:

- Ask yourself the question: would I do/not do this for every patient?

This is a key question to establish whether you are in jeopardy of being unprofessional. If you would do or not do something for every single patient, then the chances are that you are maintaining your professionalism. If the answer is no, and it is only this patient, then consider the following questions:

- Why are you doing or not doing something for this particular patient?
- Do you have a particular like or dislike for this patient?
- Consider diversity and inclusion—ask if your practice is inclusive.
- Consider your own diversity and the impact this can have on interactions with others.
- Ask: am I following the code?

4 | NOTES ON RAISING CONCERNS IDENTIFYING UNPROFESSIONALISM

CASE STUDY

David is a registered nurse working in an outpatient department, and he sees a patient in the clinic room who asks for a treatment that they do not meet the criteria for. David explains to this patient why they are unable to have this treatment and offers them the option of talking this through with a more senior colleague. This patient then becomes angry and starts raising his voice, telling David that he is not helping them and that he is useless at his job. David feels upset that he is being spoken to like this and takes the comments personally, as he feels that he has been doing his best to help the patient.

How would you maintain your professionalism if you were in David's situation?

_____
_____
_____
_____
_____
_____

TIPS

Tips for reflective practice around professionalism:

- Reflect regularly so that it becomes a natural part of your practice.
- You could build in mini-reflections, such as the end of each shift or the end of each week, to help get into the reflective practice mindset.
- For mini-reflections, could you write a couple of sentences around what you are most proud of from the week/shift?

Continued

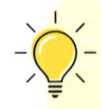

> **TIPS—cont'd**
> - For deeper reflections, look at various models of reflection to help you structure your thoughts.
> - Reflect as you go along; it's amazing what you won't remember. Even a significant event that you think you will remember the details can get lost. Reflecting at the time and then reflecting again a short time later can be a useful exercise to do. At the time, we can be caught up in emotions, but it is important to take the time to acknowledge this. When reflecting again later, we can feel completely different about the situation, and again, it is important to recognise this.
> - Consider keeping a reflective journal so that you can record events as they happen and go back and review your previous reflections so you can see how you have developed over time.
> - Always consider if you would do things differently in the future; if you wouldn't, then why not? And if yes, be specific about what you would do and how you could ensure that you will do that.

There may be times when challenging someone's conduct that you feel able to be direct and state it as it is, and there will be times when it will not be as comfortable to challenge in this way. When challenging unprofessional behaviour, consider using questions to help the person explore why they did what they did and show you are interested in hearing their view; for example:

'I notice that you did X—what made you choose this course of action?'

'I overheard you speaking to patient Y and heard you say don't be stupid; there is nothing wrong with you—what were you hoping for here?'

If you have witnessed something unprofessional and choose not to challenge or take this further, remember this quote from Lieutenant-General David Morrison:

'The standard you walk past is the standard you accept'.

(Vivid2 2021)

4 | NOTES ON RAISING CONCERNS IDENTIFYING UNPROFESSIONALISM

> There will be times when you witness a colleague behaving in an unprofessional manner. How would you challenge a colleague if you are witnessing them behaving in this way? Reflect on what you might do, how you might feel and how you would manage these feelings.
>
> Tips for challenging unprofessional behaviour:
>
> - Always speak out; the person themselves may not realise what they are doing and may be grateful for having an increased awareness of their behaviour.
> - If you feel unable to speak directly to the person themself, then speak to another colleague for support. This may be speaking to your manager or their manager.
> - If a colleague or manager advises 'that's just how they are', don't let this stop you from discussing or taking this further. Lots of cases where harm has been deliberately caused to patients have come from colleagues being complicit with unacceptable behaviour that may have been viewed as a minor issue initially and then developed into more and more unprofessional behaviour.

WHAT DOES NOT BEING PROFESSIONAL LOOK LIKE?

Throughout this book, there are many different definitions of professionalism that can be incredibly difficult to define, and it is a subjective concept. The NMC's enabling professionalism document (n.d.) states, 'Professionalism means something to everyone who works as a nurse or midwife'. Not being professional is equally as subjective yet not so tricky to define; in its most simplistic form, it can be described as "not showing the standard of behaviour or skill that is expected of a person in a skilled job' (Cambridge Dictionary 2023) However, think about your own definition of what professionalism looks like, and then think about what it doesn't look like—you would not be alone in finding the unprofessional behaviours and attitudes easier to bring to mind.

> 'As I write this, I am approaching the 42nd anniversary of becoming a registered nurse. In that time professionalism and unprofessionalism have altered. As a staff nurse, I was expected to be wearing a clean, pressed uniform each day. My hair would be "well kept", and tattoos, for example, were very much frowned on. There was a reliance on unquestioning obedience to any rules and regulations. I was once selected to be offered a free weekend (a gift from a grateful patient) because I was by then married. The director of nursing was not going to send an unmarried couple'.
>
> **Philip Ball, registered nurse and freedom to speak up guardian**

SOCIAL MEDIA POST: FACEBOOK

I'm old and retired now, but unprofessionalism to me, it's not being aware that others have so much experience and can help us in our roles despite not being nurses. For example, I learned so much about patient care and infection control from my ward domestics. I learned so many skills in patient communication and organisation from the clinical support workers. I learned to listen to my gut feelings and understand that tacit knowledge is as valuable as book learning from medics. I think sometimes there can be a them and us mentality—even between different specialisms in nursing. Not realising everyone is a valuable and necessary member of the team is unprofessional to me anyway.

I also hate patients being called bed blockers or bed nine with the dodgy kidneys. I hate tons of makeup, false nails, tons of jewellery and generally looking like you're nightclubbing. Sadly I'm a regular patient now and the last nurse I saw had so much glitter eyeshadow and I am still finding it. I'm not saying don't look after yourself and be groomed, but no one needs stick-on eyelashes to nurse. And my biggest thing is long hair worn down. I know the uniform isn't exactly glam. But still! Put yer bloody hair up. My end annoyance is walking into hospital with nurses out the front smoking in uniform.

Debbie McKinnon, retired nurse

4 | NOTES ON RAISING CONCERNS IDENTIFYING UNPROFESSIONALISM

> **SOCIAL MEDIA POST: FACEBOOK**
>
> Professionalism has changed for me over the years. I started by being smart, having my name badge on and always introducing myself as Joanne, a 1/2/3rd year student nurse. I always listened. I never argued with my seniors and learned as much as I could.
>
> Thirty-five years later, I have developed strong values and purpose. I share this with anyone who would like to chat through it, and ultimately, if we feel valued, we will allow ourselves to be vulnerable and open to new experiences.
>
> Professionalism grows as we grow. It encompasses everything, our ethics, knowledge, leadership, comportment and our identity.
>
> Joanne Bosanquet, registered nurse

Societal norms have altered over time, and nursing itself has also changed. We have become a professional body that has learnt to challenge what has gone before. Once, a 'professional' was expected to obey and be part of a cohesive group whose members acted and thought in similar ways, often because of regimented training. Now teams can be diverse and working better when individual members are recognised for their strengths, which enhances the resulting performance overall. In sports, though, unprofessional behaviour can be sanctioned immediately. That is not always possible in healthcare. It is important, therefore, that when experiencing what we think is unprofessional behaviour, we can be confident about how to report it and call it out. Freedom to speak up (explored later in this chapter) is one of the routes to do this, but not the only one.

> 'Unprofessionalism to me is not following the code of conduct as a trainee nursing associate. Standards have to be set; if it is not set, then you are allowing and promoting bad practice which could be detrimental to the people you look after. Unprofessionalism could be refusing to do a task that has been asked of you, abusing your position,

Continued

> taking more breaks than others, not helping when needed, being disruptive and generally not being accountable for any actions'.
>
> **Tanya Heath, second-year trainee nursing associate**
>
> 'To me, unprofessionalism means not following procedures, behaving or acting in a way that doesn't meet the accepted standards and not willing to change or take on board constructive criticism. Unprofessionalism is being careless, inappropriate, or not following ethical standards'.
>
> **Kafia Mohamoud, first-year trainee nursing associate**

It's important to understand that our behaviour at work can cause difficulty if expectations are not met. A simple example may be how you answer the phone: to just say 'yes' does not help the caller know who or where they have reached and can come across as unprofessional. It is important to always reassure the person which department they have gotten through to and the role of the person who answered, as people calling health and care settings are often worried and unsure, and this can help to put them at ease and save time in the long run. Another example is speaking over a patient; this is regarded as poor behaviour. As health and care professionals, we are dealing with people who have interests and expectations that they will be treated with respect.

> **TIPS**
>
> Don't forgo any conversations about the night before around patients; instead, include the patient:
>
> Get to know a little bit about all the people you care for, so you can perhaps comment on football scores, places they know or came from or who was important in their lives. This gives grounds for a common conversation.

WHEN BEING UNPROFESSIONAL BECOMES MISCONDUCT

Being unprofessional should always be taken seriously, but there are certain aspects of unprofessionalism that cross a line and become misconduct. The NMC states that 'if nurses, midwives or nursing associates fall short of the Code, what they did or failed to do may be serious professional misconduct' (NMC 2021), and this can be when there are clinical concerns that lead to harm being caused.

The NMC, when investigating misconduct, breaks concerns into three broad categories:

- Serious concerns which are more difficult to put right, for example, but not limited to:
  - breaching the professional duty of candour
  - engaging in discriminatory behaviours
  - concerns relating to harassment, including sexual harassment
  - sexual assault or relationships with patients
  - accessing, viewing or other involvement of images or videos involving child sexual abuse
  - deliberately causing harm to patients
- Serious concerns which could result in harm to patients if not put right, for example, but not limited to:
  - failure to uphold people's dignity; treat them with kindness, respect and compassion; deliver treatment care or assistance without undue delay or deliver the fundamentals of care
  - the nurse, nursing associate or midwife has not maintained the knowledge and skills for safe and effective practice.
  - there has been a failure to recognise and work within the limits of competence, accurately assess signs of normal or worsening physical or mental health, or make timely and appropriate referrals where needed.
  - there has been a failure to act without delay if they believe there is a risk to patient safety or public protection
  - there has been a failure to uphold the reputation of the profession

- Serious concerns based on the need to promote public confidence in nurses, midwives and nursing associates, for example, but not limited to:
  - if the clinical failings suggest an underlying issue with the nurse, midwife or nursing associate's attitude to people in their care.

(Adapted from How We Determine Seriousness, NMC 2024)

It's important to stress that the NMC always looks carefully at the context and background of each individual case reported to them as misconduct, as sometimes misconduct is as a result of organisational or system failures.

> **CASE STUDY**
>
> Rose is a registered nurse who works in a care home. Often she is the only registered nurse on duty and is responsible for 65 residents. One morning, Rose arrives, and she is the only registered nurse on duty. She starts the morning medication round. After 20 minutes, there is an emergency with one of the residents which Rose has to attend to, and this takes a considerable amount of time, after which she returns to the medication round. Rose feels under pressure to administer medications quickly. The next day, Rose arrives for duty, and her manager pulls her to one side and explains that she had made a medication error the previous day. Rose and her manager discuss and reflect on the medication error and start to look at the context in which the error was made. Rose understands that, ultimately, the medication error is her responsibility, and expresses this to her manager. However, both the manager and Rose agree that the needs of the residents far outweigh what one registered nurse is able to provide and that staffing levels need to be adjusted. Rose and her manager were able to see how circumstances had led to the medication error.

Another aspect of unprofessionalism is the deliberate action taken that ends in harm to a patient or colleague. Of course, this is taken very seriously by the NMC and is covered by the code of conduct and the criminal law if required. Sadly, examples exist even in 2024.

THE BRISTOL BABY SCANDAL

In the late 1990s, Bristol hit the headlines, as 30–35 children at the Bristol Royal Infirmary (BRI) who underwent heart surgery had died, and it was reported that they probably would have survived if they were treated elsewhere. An article written at the time stated, 'These "excess" deaths took place in a unit where mortality at the time for children aged under 1 was probably double that for England as a whole, and even higher for neonates. Around a third of children who underwent open heart surgery received less than adequate care' (Dyer 2001). The inquiry report stated that the system of care was flawed and there was poor teamwork between professionals. The failings at Bristol were not just down to the surgeons alone; the inquiry showed inadequacies at every point, including referral, diagnosis, surgery and intensive care (Dyer 2001). Michelle Samson provides an account of the events from her perspective.

> 'In the last year of my training, I switched to a different trust, and I had a two-month placement on a cardiac surgery unit for children and adults. The atmosphere on the unit was very strange and I noticed several members of the nursing team would regularly be in tears. I also noticed one member of the multi-disciplinary team appeared to be treated differently to everyone else and there was tangible tension between him and the rest of the team. Although I learnt a lot on this placement, I was very relieved when my placement ended due to the weird atmosphere on the unit. The year after I left the unit the Bristol baby heart scandal hit the press; I will never forget the image of tiny coffins outside the hospital when the bereaved families protested. This is when I realised what had been happening on the unit and why the team were so emotional; I also realised that the member of the team who was ostracised and ignored was the person who had raised concerns about the unacceptable mortality rate.

Continued

Dr. Stephen Bolsin was the anaesthetist who became very concerned about the mortality rate of babies having cardiac surgery at the BRI. Data during 1984–1995 demonstrated a 50% higher mortality rate for certain cardiac surgery for babies and children. If this information had been given to parents when they were making the decision about whether to go ahead with surgery, I imagine they may have made a different decision and would have requested surgery elsewhere. Dr. Bolsin was not supported by senior managers at the BRI, so he whistle blew to the press and this led to one of the biggest public inquiries in NHS history. Below is a quote from the latter report which has always resonated with me:

> *"The culture of the future must be a culture of safety and of quality; a culture of openness and of accountability; a culture of public service; a culture in which collaborative teamwork is prized; and a culture of flexibility in which innovation can flourish in response to patients' needs."*

Dr. Bolsin felt he couldn't continue practising in the United Kingdom, so (he) relocated to Australia where he is head of patient safety at a large hospital; the huge difference he made to patient safety in the United Kingdom was recognised when he received the Royal College of Anaesthetists medal for promoting safety in anaesthesia.

Several changes happened as a result of the inquiries, including the change that clinicians were encouraged to discuss risks in services and how those risk could be mitigated. During these speciality meetings, patients who had come to harm or had died were discussed to explore if things could have been done differently and if there was any learning to take forward.

This was all happening in my first year as a registered nurse; I started to hear words such as governance and whistleblowing, and a

> *theoretical shift was made towards being open and transparent. In my career, I have to say, I didn't really feel or see this until many years later when I was a senior nurse in the community and huge concerns were raised about poor care and much higher-than-expected mortality rate at the Mid Staffordshire NHS Foundation Trust'.*
>
> **Michelle Samson, registered nurse and service delivery lead**

THE REPORT OF THE MID STAFFORDSHIRE NHS FOUNDATION TRUST INQUIRY

The report of the Mid Staffordshire NHS Foundation Trust Public Inquiry was published on 6 February 2013, and it examined the causes of the failings in care at Mid Staffordshire NHS Foundation Trust between 2005 and 2009. Robert Francis (2013), who chaired the inquiry, states, regarding Mid Staffordshire, that the investigation into the care provided by the Mid Staffordshire NHS Foundation Trust came about because of rising concerns around mortality rates and how the investigation caused considerable public and political concern. Francis explains how the experiences of over 900 people were collected in the report, giving a voice to patients, their families and staff. Francis (2013) outlines how the report told many stories that were hard to hear:

- A whistleblowing nurse in the accident and emergency department was not protected from harassment by colleagues of the staff whose conduct she had reported, to the extent that she did not feel safe to leave work at night unaccompanied.
- A shortage of nursing staff and inadequate skill mix was identified, but remedial action took far too long. In the meantime, little consideration appears to have been given to the patient safety implications.
- A reluctance to engage with or in management was widespread among professional staff.

- Clinical audit and other governance measures were, at best, approached reluctantly by many.
- Above all, so many examples of appalling nursing care and attention could not have occurred if medical staff and senior nurses had looked out for and corrected the deficiencies that were so obvious to patients and those close to them'.

Francis (2013) identifies reasons why the failures came about:

Self-interest: Clinicians were afraid to raise concerns because of the possibility of adverse consequences for their careers or pay.

Fear: Staff members were afraid of raising concerns because of the potential reaction from colleagues. Patients were afraid to complain, as they were fearful of retribution from the people caring for them.

Isolation: Clinicians in some disciplines were isolated and did not participate in peer networks.

Tolerance of poor standards: The environment at Mid Staffordshire was so stressful, understaffed and underresourced that staff began to accept poor standards.

Lack of leadership: An example of this was the passive way in which the report from the Royal College of Surgeons was received at Mid Staffordshire, with very little effective action taking place to resolve issues.

There were 129 recommendations; the report talked about a culture of openness and transparency, putting the patient first.

Debra Hazeldine MBE, daughter of deceased Ellen Linstead, who was a patient at Mid Staffordshire NHS Foundation Trust tells, her story.

> 'MidStaffs, my family's reality.
>
> In 2006 I became a patient safety campaigner without even knowing it. I didn't ever want to be a patient safety campaigner. I was very happy and content with the life I had.
>
> From 2005 to 2009, between 400 and 600 more patients died at Mid Staffordshire Hospital than would have been expected. The high mortality data being a red flag to go and check. To actually open a

door, enter the ward and see and hear the patients and their families' experiences, enter the ward and you could actually see and hear and smell the suffering. Cost cutting and prioritising of targets and obtaining Foundation Trust status sadly resulted in the patients and families becoming lost and not always a priority in a care system that had, in parts, become immune to the sound of pain.

The public inquiry heard from many witnesses and over a million pages of documentary material. A "story of the unnecessary suffering of hundreds of people." A lack of care, compassion, humanity and leadership. The most basic standards of care were not observed. I was one of those witnesses that gave evidence on oath in public, trying to give my dead mum a voice. The voice she no longer had but desperately needed.

A report to the majority, something that happened to other people. One of those "other people" was my mum, Ellen Linstead. My lovely mum died an avoidable death in heartbreaking circumstances in MidStaffs in 2006, aged just 67. A small district general hospital in the West Midlands. From the outside it looked like any other district general hospital. Somewhere people pass every day going about their busy lives.

If I may, I will take you back to just some of the most painful memories I have, in the hope that this will explain exactly why I campaigned for so many, many long exhausting emotional years. Some of this was happening whilst my mum was continually being told that there was no clinical reason for her to be in hospital and she simply needed to put more effort into her physio. She was labelled a "bed blocker". My Mum sat and cried, she just wanted to go home.

On one occasion even before I entered the ward, I could hear my mum screaming. Please stop for a second and try and imagine that this was your loved one, your Mum screaming out in so much pain. I could never become immune to the sound of my lovely Mum in terrible pain. I literally dropped my bag, and I ran to her. She was half on the floor and half on a commode, and she grabbed my hand and said, "Please

Continued

Deb, don't let me die in here!" Our eyes met; the look of utter despair on my mum's face to this day never leaves me. I categorically failed her, failed to be able to keep her safe as she had done for me my entire childhood. To this day this haunts my every waking and sleeping hour. I let her down when she needed me the most.

Whilst my mum was trying to complete her physiotherapy, I would hold her as she cried and stated that she was in pain in her back and her ribs. She was told that the pain was all in her head, and she should put more effort into her physio and becoming mobile. Because somebody else needed that bed she was occupying, again my mum was labelled a bed blocker. This distressed her so much because she tried so very hard to become mobile. It wasn't until after her death that I read in her notes that she had preventable falls in hospital and had fractures in her back and ribs. You see the pain was not just in her head. I asked if I could take my mum to another hospital, take her home and I was told, "If you discharge your Mum and she dies, you are responsible".

Throughout the day myself, my dad or my brother would need to be with my mum to support with food and fluids. I took in food, fluids and blankets. The call button was always out of reach, food and fluids out of reach, compassion and empathy out of reach. My mum's legs were so sore from being left sitting in urine-soaked sheets for so long that the skin was peeling off. The window next to my mum was broken and would not shut. A nurse kindly tried to stuff a sheet at the window to stop the icy winter air from coming in. When I was visiting one day, my mum was so cold; I took off my thick woollen cardigan and put it on her, I left it on her. My Mum was concerned that I would become cold on the journey home, always concerned for her daughter.

On another occasion I was sitting with my mum at visiting time, and faeces just fell from her and covered her, the floor and the chair she was sitting on. My Mum was mortified and quietly began to cry. I searched for staff to support and there was no one. In the end I got down on my hands and knees with paper towels and began to try and clean her. C-Diff in all its glory for all to see and smell. No dignity, no support.

On a Sunday afternoon in December, the light was fading fast. I sat in the corner of my mum's room as she was feeling unwell; I was so worried to leave her. She was half asleep and feeling very sick. Suddenly a member of staff came into the room; I'm not sure if they saw me; they didn't acknowledge how poorly my mum was looking and feeling. This member of staff shouted at my mum, wanting to know what medication she had taken that day. My mum jolted awake and did not respond because she was half asleep; the member of staff shouted again. The despair in my mum's eyes once again. This member of staff stated sharply that you should be aware of what medication you have taken. I stood up at this point, and the member of staff looked startled at me being there and swiftly left the room. My mum put her arm out. "Don't say anything Deb; I'm worried what will happen". I rubbed my mum's arm and tried to reassure her and said, "Don't worry, maybe I can answer their questions, try not to worry, Mum."

As I left the room, I was filled with utter despair as I called after the member of staff, asking if I could help, could I try and answer your questions?

The grade 4 pressure sores that my mum developed over time left me feeling despair again at the pain they must have been causing her.

Trying to speak out in a clinical setting when you are labelled as an overprotective daughter who is just so worried about leaving her Mum alone is mortifying. The consultant had to write in the notes that I could visit at any time to support my mum, the support she desperately needed and because of the abuse I received. Hearing someone say doesn't she know the damn visiting times when I was so worried about my mum crushes you as a person. Trying to speak out as a patient in a clinical setting, in your nightclothes, when feeling vulnerable and unwell is incredibly scary and can feel impossible. I had so many sleepless nights worrying what happens to those who have no one, only the

Continued

system to be their advocate when they are most vulnerable, trying to be heard, when the system had lost sight of the patients. I fear my mum died thinking many did not care. A few days before my mum's death, we were told the devastating news that she was going to die. Not in a private room, not in a quiet setting where we could try and absorb this horrific information but in a corridor, as we were told that there were no rooms available.

After my mum's death, we thought the worst had happened and the despair we felt could not increase further, and then it just did. We, as a family, were told that we would not be able to view my mum at the undertaker's because of all the hospital-acquired infections that she had. I desperately needed to see my mum out of that hospital setting, even if only for a few moments, and I begged to be able to do so. I saw my mum briefly, and my final memories are of her head protruding from a body bag. I was unable to hold her hand or kiss her forehead gently, but I needed to be with her to the very end, however bad it got. I needed to be able to say, "I'm so sorry I couldn't keep you safe, I was so sorry I let you down".

We were given my mum's belongings back to us in a bin bag covered in faeces. Her dressing gown, which we had been told had gone for cleaning, her glasses, clothes all covered in faeces, all needing to be thrown away. Painful memories to carry with me always. Then my mum was returned to us in a waste bag marked toxic.

It should never have taken a small group of bereaved relatives campaigning in the wind, ice, rain and snow over many emotionally exhausting years to be heard and the truth exposed for all to see clearly. Because, in my humble opinion, if your washer can't be repaired, you may find yourself needing to complain, but if your mum has suffered unnecessarily before dying and should not have, raising this, speaking out is not complaining. I should never have needed to give evidence to the healthcare commission, independent inquiry and on oath at the public inquiry, but how would I ever have any peace if I did not try? Desperately try to ensure that no other mothers and daughters had our dreadful final harrowing memories. To this day my mum remains my first thoughts on waking and my last thoughts before sleeping. We were always more than our final memories; however, those final memories remain most prominent.

Some desperately tried to make Mid Staffordshire simply about numbers, disagreeing about how many people had or had not lost their lives. When, in fact, MidStaffs was primarily about mothers, fathers, sisters, sons, daughters, brothers, aunts, uncles, friends and neighbours, their last weeks, days, hours. Precious time they had hoped to be spending with their loved ones, stopped in its tracks, suddenly unnecessarily suffering before going from a unit number to a deceased unit number. Within the Mid Staffordshire reports, enclosed in the pages is so much learning and very important to always remember it is a precious loved one's final days. It was the bereaved families' lives yesterday; it will be today and tomorrow.

Death comes to all; it's how you die and the memories you leave with loved ones for eternity.

You can't possibly remember every patient and family you come into contact with, but I promise you, they will remember you. You are there at the most emotional times in our lives. In our moments of celebration and joy and in our saddest moments. When we come into this world and when we leave.

Compassion, empathy, caring for others begins with caring for yourselves, and I believe that begins with teaching. Creating in training the culture that it is necessary to look after yourself, take care of your own health and well-being and that of your fellow students and colleagues. To try and avoid the toxic culture of stress and becoming immune to the sound of pain; that was the reality for some in Mid Staffordshire. How can healthcare professionals be held responsible or held to account if systems are not supporting them to deliver the safe standard of care that I absolutely believe they wish to give their patients? Compassion and empathy fatigue do not happen overnight,

Continued

> *and they have a devastating impact on patients, families and staff. If NHS systems are not focused on supporting staff, patients and families, they are simply losing sight of the most important people. We all need clinical support at some point in our lives; none of us should ever feel that we don't matter because we all matter to someone. I've said many times that the NHS's best asset is its dedicated staff. We as a nation depend on you so much and we always will. Thank you for the positive difference you are going to make in our lives'.*
>
> **Debra Hazeldine, daughter of deceased, Ellen Linstead.**

Having read Debra Hazeldine's account of her mum's experience of Mid Staffordshire, think about what you can do to ensure that you make a positive difference to the people you care for:

_____

_____

_____

_____

_____

A year after the Mid Staffordshire NHS Foundation Trust Inquiry Report, 'Culture change in the NHS, applying the lessons of The Francis Report' (2015) was published, which called for action across six core themes:

- Culture
- Compassionate care
- Leadership
- Standards
- Openness, transparency
- Duty of candour

4 | NOTES ON RAISING CONCERNS IDENTIFYING UNPROFESSIONALISM

> 'For me in my practise as a senior nurse, the most important elements of the Mid Staffordshire NHS Foundation Trust Inquiry Report were openness, transparency and candour. Raising a concern is part of this being able to say when things aren't right and if we fall below the standards we say we will maintain. Working in this way allows me to be authentic and transparent and this aligns to my core values. I am a compassionate leader committed to healthcare being delivered in a transparent, open way with candour, allowing me to work in a compassionate way.
>
> This report is probably been the most pivotal report in my nursing career, and I would say probably one where the recommendations were put in place in quite a fast pace, and looking back, some of the things, like duty of candour or freedom to speak with and whistleblowing, have become something that's discussed in daily practise. I don't think I've seen any instances in the last decade where duty of candour wasn't considered immediately; clinical teams speaking to patients and their families in an authentic way with candour and clarity has become normal business as usual. I will never forget the pictures of all the people who had died due to neglect and mistreatment at Mid Staffordshire.
>
> Although raising a concern can feel overwhelming or scary, there are processes within every NHS trust and healthcare organisation to make this easier. Freedom to speak up guardians are available to speak to people that have concerns and signpost and support them. All concerns are confidential, but the NHS trust/organisation board is aware of any concerns that are raised, and the organisation has to report publicly how many concerns have been raised'.
>
> **Michelle Samson, registered nurse and service delivery lead**

Robert Francis was subsequently asked to chair the inquiry into the Mid Staffordshire Hospital that resulted in him recommending that staff should have an independent place and person to go to where they could raise their concerns. Out of this, the government of the day set up the National Guardian Office, (NGO) and mandated all NHS acute trusts to have freedom to speak up guardians in 2016.

RAISING CONCERNS

There were staff members at Mid Staffordshire who tried to speak up and experienced controlling and bullying behaviour from colleagues. These controlling or bullying behaviours can be outside the values of the organisation you are placed in. Fig. 4.1 outlines bullying behaviours (adapted from NHS Scotland 2010):

There are many routes for reporting what can be described as unprofessional behaviour. Fig. 4.2 explores a few of them.

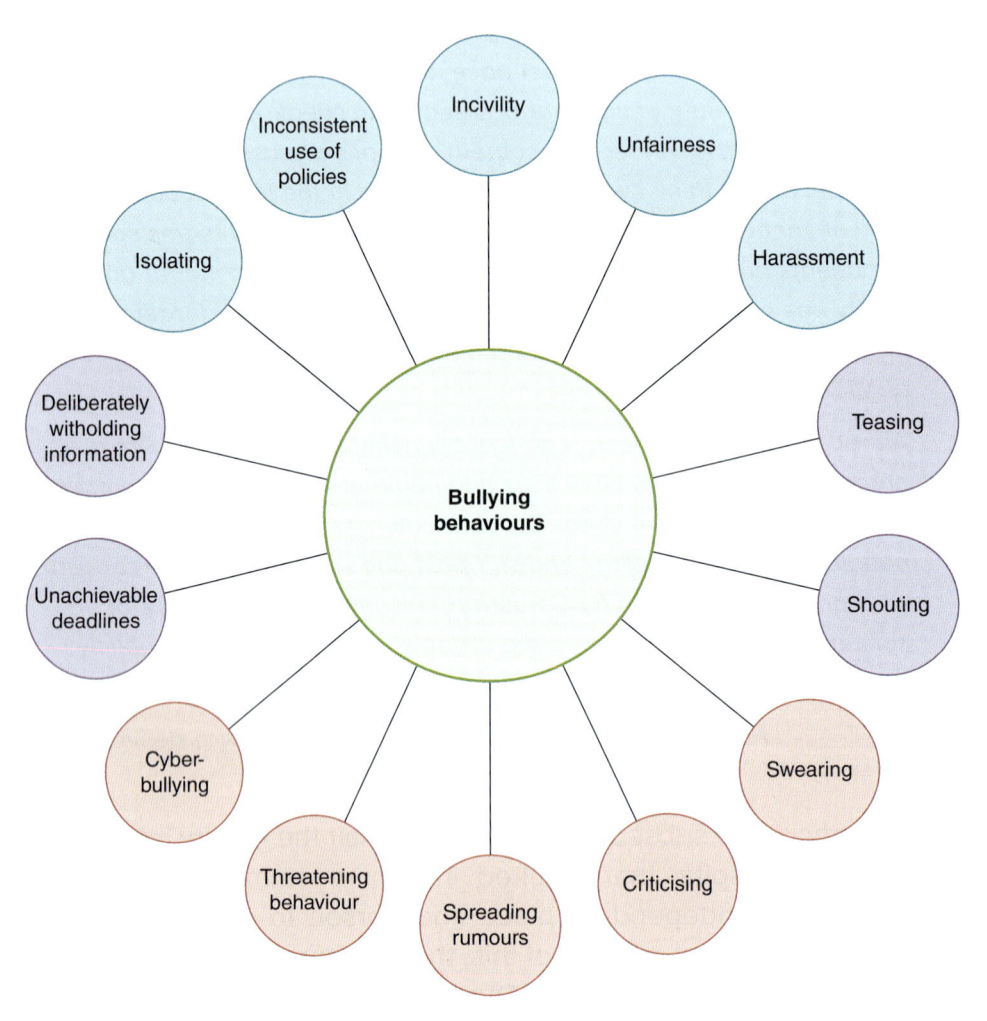

Figure 4.1 Bullying behaviours. Adapted from NHS Scotland 2010.

4 | NOTES ON RAISING CONCERNS IDENTIFYING UNPROFESSIONALISM

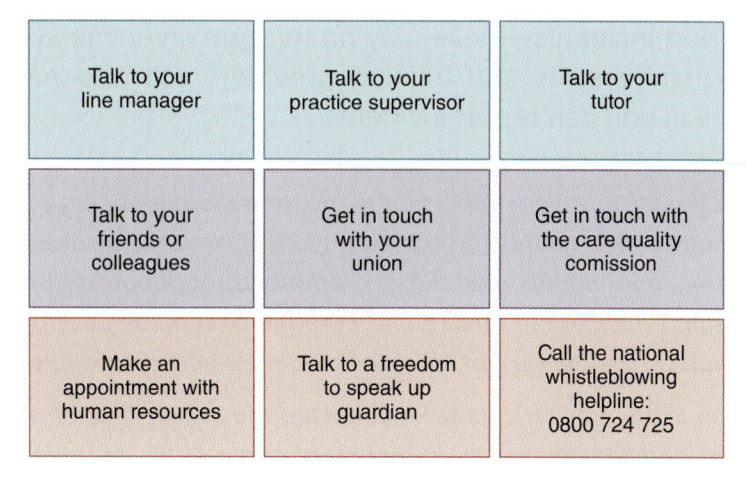

Talk to your line manager	Talk to your practice supervisor	Talk to your tutor
Talk to your friends or colleagues	Get in touch with your union	Get in touch with the care quality comission
Make an appointment with human resources	Talk to a freedom to speak up guardian	Call the national whistleblowing helpline: 0800 724 725

Figure 4.2   Routes of reporting unprofessional behaviour.

However, all NHS organisations are expected to have freedom to speak up guardians. 'Freedom to Speak Up is about encouraging a positive culture where people feel they can speak up and their voices will be heard, and their suggestions acted upon', and freedom to speak up guardians are 'an alternative route to normal channels for speaking up such as via line managers', supporting people to raise concerns (Health Education England n.d.).

> *'As a guardian, I rarely hear about direct clinical concerns, as there are many quicker ways to report concerns, especially about patients. These are important to understand as a student or trainee, so you can be confident of who to tell about a concern. There can be other areas where you think the behaviour I am experiencing or witnessing is not acceptable. I hear more about when someone thinks they are being treated badly in some way by a line manager or colleague'.*
>
> **Philip Ball, registered nurse and freedom to speak up guardian**

It's vital to understand, as a health and care professional, that silence isn't safe. If any of us witness something that does not feel right, we should report it. The organisations where we learn and work will have ways to report incidents—these may be through an online system such as RADAR. Universities and training providers will also have routes through which you can report incidents.

> *'Professionalism is very important to me, and I feel that I have personally delivered this throughout my 29-year nursing career. A belief in lifelong learning has meant that a priority throughout has been accessing education to ensure that I am the best nurse possible. This has enabled the delivery of safe and evidence-based care to patients.*
>
> *Early on in my nursing career I recognised the importance of raising a concern and very much felt, as a student nurse, I was an advocate for patients, especially if they are unable to speak and give their view themself.*
>
> *One of the nursing placements I had in the second year of my training was in a local nursing home; myself and two other students had a 4-week placement there. A couple of things happened in the first week that I felt very uncomfortable with, and I raised concerns with the matron of the home and the university where I was doing my nurse training. Here are three examples of things that happened in the first few days of the placement.*
>
> 1. *Two ladies were living in a shared room. I arrived in their room, and one lady was in the middle of the room on a commode having her bowels open when a tray with her breakfast was put in front of her. The second lady was in her chair sitting in front of the lady on the commode; she had a tray with her breakfast on it. Unsurprisingly, neither lady was able to eat their breakfast. I spoke to the care assistants and said, "Shall we move the lady on the commode to the ensuite bathroom and bring both ladies breakfasts back later?" This was met with a look of surprise.*
> 2. *A gentleman sitting in the lounge asked to go to the toilet. I said, "Of course." As I was getting him ready to go to the toilet, I was told I couldn't take him now because people are toileted in order of how they are seated in the lounge. I expressed that he was one of the few people that had bladder sensation, and I wanted to keep that intact, so I needed to take him to the toilet now. I went to look*

at where the toilet was and was shocked to see one lady stood in the hall naked from the waist down with a care assistant and another lady sat on the toilet with the door open in full view on the front door and hall. I was horrified and asked the staff what they were doing, and they said they always did it like this. I asked if they would like to be toileted in the same manner, and I had blank stares. I expressed my concern that this was a complete lack of privacy and dignity, and I would bring it up with the matron.

3. *I returned to the lounge, and a lady asked me to close the curtains, as the sun was in her face. I said, "Of course," and immediately closed the curtains. At this point, the matron entered the room and shouted at me for closing the curtains and demanded I open them immediately. I explained I couldn't do so because the sun was hurting the lady's eyes, hence why I shut the curtains; she shouted at me to open them, and I said, "I'm afraid I can't do that". I was summoned to her office, and the matron proceeded to tell me off for disobeying her orders. I explained I was perplexed that she wanted the curtains open when it was doing harm to a lady. I said I had other things that had concerned me and told her about the other scenarios. After a very unpleasant meeting, she told me I had to change my attitude; I told her I was going to contact my university and would be making a formal a statement of concern about the home. The university tutor came to the home, and all the students were told to leave. The home was taken off the list of placements for students. I did make a formal concern to the council, and the home was inspected and required serious improvement.*

It was a rather dramatic introduction to raising concerns for me, but I felt very strongly the people living there deserved much better care. Many of them had dementia and were unable to raise concerns, so I felt very much obliged to do so on their behalf. I still feel as passionately about this over 30 years later'.

Michelle Samson, registered nurse and service delivery lead

In 2023, the NMC produced guidance on raising concerns, 'Raising concerns: Guidance for nurses, midwives and nursing associates', which includes advice for nursing students raising concerns. The NMC (2023) states that the principles of 'Raising concerns: Guidance for nurses, midwives and nursing associates' also apply to student nurses, midwives and nursing associates, and they suggest the following action should you need to raise concerns:

- Nursing students should inform their mentor, tutor or lecturer immediately if they believe that they, a colleague or anyone else may be putting someone at risk of harm.
- Nursing students should seek help immediately from an appropriately qualified professional if someone they are providing care for has suffered harm for any reason.
- Nursing students should seek help from their mentor, tutor or lecturer if people disclose that they are unhappy about their care or treatment.

The NMC (2023) states that they recognise that it might not be easy for nursing students to raise a concern; they may not be sure what to do, or the process may seem quite daunting. The NMC stresses that if nursing students want some advice at any stage, they recommend that they talk to their university tutor or lecturer, their mentor or another registered nurse, midwife or nursing associate. Nursing students can also speak to their professional body, trade union or Protect (Protect provides free, confidential whistleblowing advice and can be found at protect-advice.org.uk).

CONCLUSION

History tells us that when concerns aren't raised, the quality of care and, ultimately, the people we care for suffer. Being a nursing student means that you must safeguard the people you care for, and safeguarding the health and well-being of those people means that they should not be exposed to abuse or neglect. There is support in place, and if you ever find yourself needing to raise a concern, think about contacting your mentor, tutor, freedom to speak up guardian or a registered nurse you trust. Even though raising concerns is hard to do, nursing students have a duty to raise concerns about professionalism if they have them.

Space for reader's own reflection:

REFERENCES

Cambridge Dictionary. 2023. Unprofessional. https://dictionary.cambridge.org/dictionary/english/unprofessional [Accessed January 18, 2024]

Dyer, C., 2001. Bristol inquiry condemns hospital's "club culture", BMJ 323.

Francis, Q.C.R., 2013. Mid Staffordshire – some reflections for clinicians. Trends Urol. Men's Health 4, 17–20.

Health Education England. n.d. Freedom to speak up guardians. https://www.hee.nhs.uk/our-work/freedom-speak-guardians [Accessed January 18, 2024]

NHS Scotland. 2010. Bullying and harassment policy: Examples of bullying behaviour. https://workforce.nhs.scot/supporting-documents/tool/bullying-and-harassment-policy-examples-of-bullying-behaviour/ [Accessed January 18, 2024]

Nursing and Midwifery Council. n.d. Enabling professionalism in nursing and midwifery practice. https://www.nmc.org.uk/globalassets/sitedocuments/other-publications/enabling-professionalism.pdf [Accessed January 18, 2024]

Nursing and Midwifery Council. 2021. Misconduct. https://www.nmc.org.uk/ftp-library/understanding-fitness-to-practise/fitness-to-practise-allegations/misconduct/ [Accessed January 18, 2024]

Nursing and Midwifery Council. 2024. 'How we determine seriousness'. https://www.nmc.org.uk/ftp-library/understanding-fitness-to-practise/how-we-determine-seriousness/ [Accessed November 12, 2024]

Nursing and Midwifery Council. 2018. Understanding fitness to practise. https://www.nmc.org.uk/ftp-library/understanding-fitness-to-practise/ [Accessed January 18, 2024]

Vivid2. 2021. Great speeches – David Morrison 'The standard you walk past...' https://vividmethod.com/leadership-message-the-standard-you-walk-past-is-the-standard-you-accept/ [Accessed January 18, 2024]

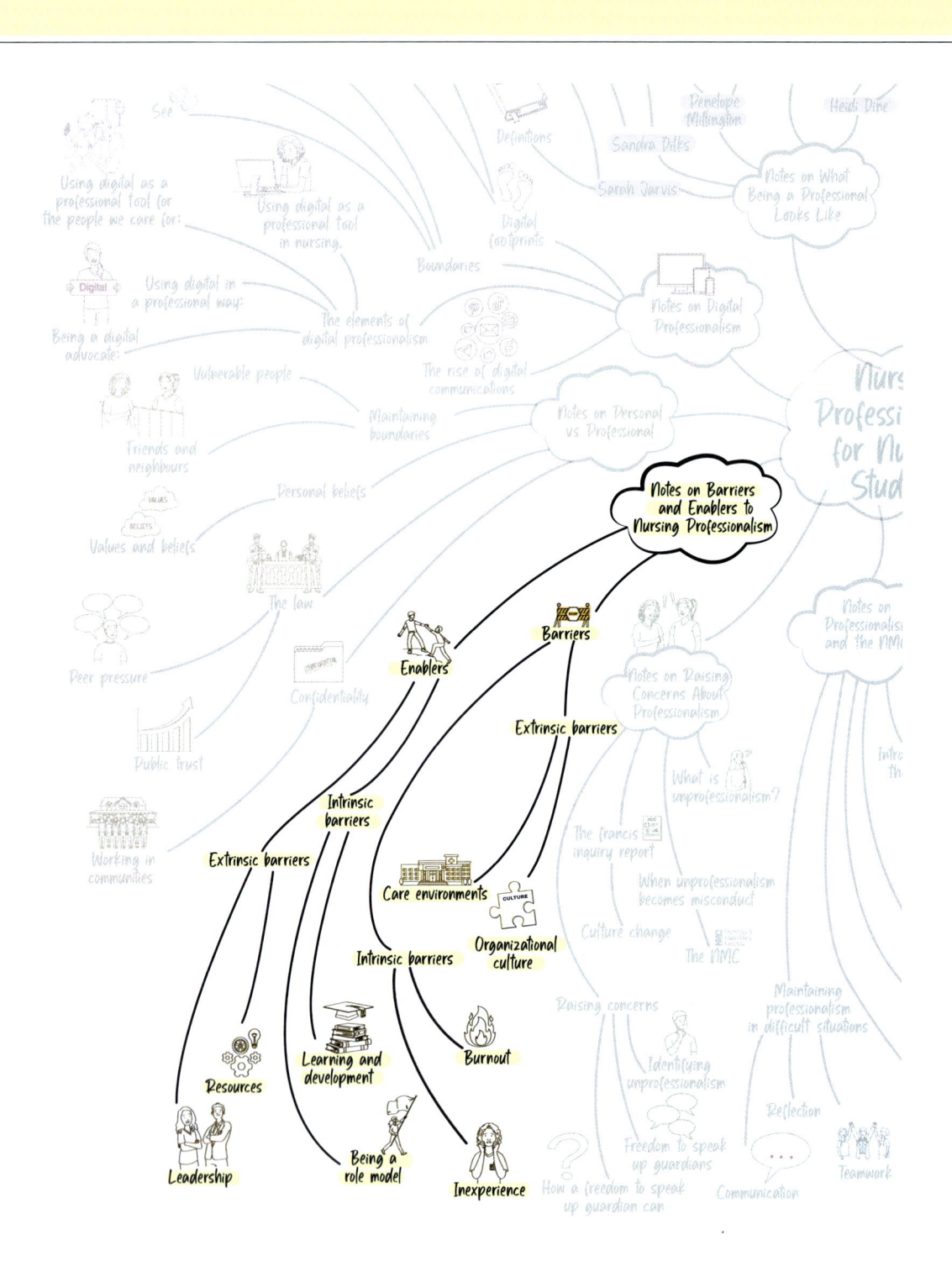

Notes on Barriers and Enablers to Nursing Professionalism

Enablers
- **Extrinsic barriers**
  - Resources
  - Leadership
- **Intrinsic barriers**
  - Learning and development
  - Being a role model

Barriers
- **Extrinsic barriers**
  - Care environments
  - Organizational culture
- **Intrinsic barriers**
  - Burnout
  - Inexperience

5

NOTES ON BARRIERS AND ENABLERS TO NURSING PROFESSIONALISM

Teresa Chinn (she/her) ■ Tara Iles (she/her)

INTRODUCTION

Nursing professionalism serves as the bedrock of quality patient care, encompassing a broad spectrum of attributes, behaviours and values that contribute to effective nursing practice. While the concept of professionalism has been extensively explored in this book, nurses and nursing students often encounter various barriers that provide challenges in maintaining and demonstrating professionalism consistently. Conversely, there are numerous enablers that facilitate the cultivation of professionalism among nurses and nursing students, thereby enhancing their practice and positively impacting patient outcomes. This chapter aims to give nursing students an awareness of those barriers and enablers, with the view that if nursing students are aware of and able to identify influences on professionalism, they will be more aware of the implications for nursing practice and patient care.

BARRIERS TO NURSING PROFESSIONALISM

Professionalism in nursing is not a static concept; it needs the right conditions in which to thrive. For nursing students, this is particularly relevant, as students will dip in and out of healthcare environments, experiencing many different cultures, leadership styles and situations.

In addition to this, nursing students are having to juggle placements, academic work and sometimes complex personal lives. All of these things can be a barrier to professionalism, and it's important that nursing students are able to understand and realise the impact that these factors have.

In a qualitative study looking at challenges to compassionate care, Babaei and Taleghani (2019) identify barriers to professionalism; these can be separated into two categories:

- Extrinsic barriers to nursing professionalism: these are barriers that relate to organisational or situational factors.
- Intrinsic barriers to nursing professionalism: these are barriers that relate to oneself, health and well-being.

While often the reality is that these barriers intertwine, this categorisation provides a great way to explore them.

A NOTE ON INTRINSIC AND EXTRINSIC

While for the purpose of this chapter, we have distinctly separated factors influencing professionalism into intrinsic and extrinsic, the reality is that often there is no distinction. Intrinsic factors influencing professionalism while discussed as being internal and the responsibility of the nurse or nursing student are heavily influenced and twisted in with extrinsic factors. Conversely, extrinsic factors could be viewed as being solely the responsibility of employers; however, when it comes to workplace cultures and environments, everyone is responsible for identifying and taking action on factors that could impact professionalism. Morrison (2021) famously said, 'The standard you walk past is the standard you accept'.

EXTRINSIC BARRIERS TO NURSING PROFESSIONALISM

Employers have a principal role to play in supporting professionalism and enabling it to flourish and develop. In regard to extrinsic barriers, employers need to be aware of supportive environments in which nurses and nursing students feel valued and the barriers to professionalism that may exist (Health and Care Professionals Council 2014). In turn, nurses and nursing students need to be aware of extrinsic barriers to professionalism and the impact that they may have on them and the care they provide.

Fig. 5.1 outlines some extrinsic barriers to professionalism as identified by Babaei and Taleghani (2019).

Care environments

The quality of care environments significantly influences nurses' and nursing students' ability to uphold professionalism. If you have ever been in a chaotic environment (whether it's a healthcare environment or not), you will know that it can compromise your ability to do your job well. In nursing, this compromise is in regard to providing patient-centred care and engaging in professional communication and collaboration (Chapman et al. 2018).

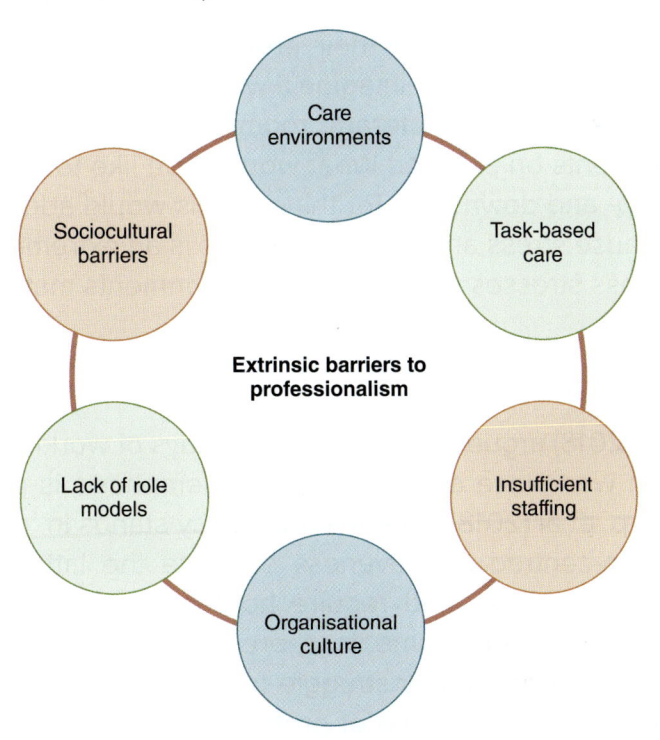

Figure 5.1 Extrinsic barriers to nursing professionalism.

> **Think about a time when you have been working in a chaotic environment (it doesn't necessarily have to be a health or nursing environment). How did the chaos affect your ability to do your job?**
>
> _____
>
> _____
>
> _____
>
> _____
>
> _____

The physical layout of care settings can also have an impact and hinder nurses' and nursing students' ability to deliver timely and effective care. This, in turn, can also affect their professionalism by placing undue pressure and stress on staff. Imagine a ward that was spread across two floors, with clinical rooms, storage rooms and nurses' stations on one floor and patients on another! What would it be like to work there, having to run up- and downstairs for things? This would add time to everything and cause stress and exhaustion. This is an extreme example, but it nevertheless stresses the point that environments matter!

Task-based care

Sharp et al. (2018) argue that task-focused ways of working can become prevalent in workplace cultures where an emphasis is placed on efficiency. Sharp. et al (2018) state that efficiency stands in 'contrast to ideals of person-centred effectiveness because the latter may actually slow down procedures and require holistic approaches, rather than segmented care'. In environments where nursing care becomes primarily task oriented, nurses may struggle to prioritise holistic patient care, leading to a diminished sense of professionalism and patient dissatisfaction (Terry et al. 2019).

Insufficient staffing

Understaffing poses a significant barrier to nursing professionalism, as it increases workload and time pressures, impeding nurses' ability to deliver safe and effective care and eroding their professional autonomy (Griffiths et al. 2018). Inadequate staffing levels not only strain nurses' physical and emotional resources but also compromise their ability to prioritise patient needs and provide the level of care they aspire to deliver.

Organisational culture

The prevailing organisational culture can either support or undermine nursing professionalism. Cultures that prioritise productivity over quality care may discourage nurses from advocating for patients' best interests and upholding professional standards (Hutchinson and Jackson 2019). Conversely, organisations that foster a culture of respect, collaboration and continuous learning empower nurses to uphold professionalism and contribute to positive patient outcomes.

Lack of role models

Role models play a crucial role in shaping professional identity and behaviour, providing guidance, inspiration and mentorship to less experienced nurses. However, in environments where role models are scarce or exhibit unprofessional conduct, nurses may struggle to emulate desired professional attributes and behaviours.

> **THE NMC SAYS**
>
> **20.8** Act as a role model of professional behaviour for students and newly qualified nurses, midwives and nursing associates to aspire to.

The absence of positive role models within the nursing workforce can hinder nurses' and nursing students' professional development and discourage them from aspiring to higher standards of practice (Elliott and Coventry 2020).

Sociocultural barriers

Sociocultural factors such as gender biases or discrimination can impact nurses' and nursing students' sense of professional identity and confidence, influencing their ability to uphold professionalism in the face of adversity (Hupcey et al. 2018). Discriminatory practices or unequal treatment within healthcare settings can undermine nurses' morale and sense of belonging, posing significant barriers to their professional development and advancement.

INTRINSIC BARRIERS TO NURSING PROFESSIONALISM

Intrinsic barriers in this sense are all about those barriers that exist on a personal level, either consciously or subconsciously; however, these barriers are hugely affected by extrinsic factors, both in the workplace and at home.

Fig. 5.2 outlines intrinsic barriers to nursing professionalism as suggested by Babaei and Taleghani (2019).

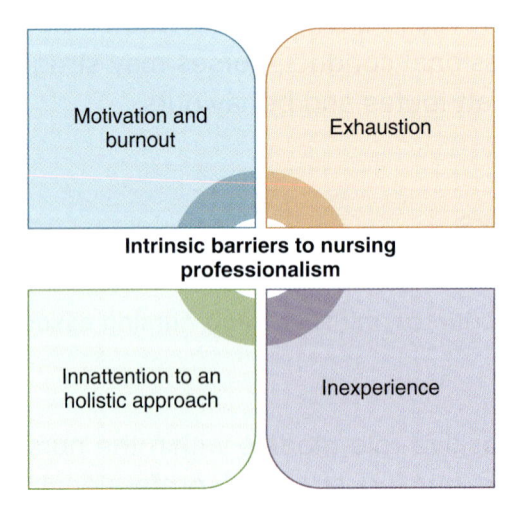

Figure 5.2 Intrinsic barriers to nursing professionalism.

5 | NOTES ON BARRIERS AND ENABLERS TO NURSING PROFESSIONALISM

Motivation and burnout

Low motivation and burnout can diminish nurses' enthusiasm for professional development and reflective practice, hindering their ability to maintain professionalism and deliver high-quality care (Jackson et al. 2020). Burnout, characterised by emotional exhaustion, depersonalisation and reduced personal accomplishment, is prevalent among healthcare professionals, including nurses, and can have detrimental effects on patient safety and care quality. Dall'Ora and Saville (2021) state that there are 'reported associations between some subscales of burnout and low job performance, sickness absence, poor general health, missed patient care and job dissatisfaction'. Therefore it is of vast importance that nurses and nursing students take care of themselves and their mental health and well-being. NHS England and NHS Improvement Midlands (n.d.) identify 11 areas in which nurses can care for themselves and some resources to help; these are summarised in the following tips.

> **TIPS**
>
> Taking care of yourself as a nurse or nursing student is very important; if you are unable to prioritise your own health and well-being, this can have an effect on your motivation and lead to burnout, which, in turn, can have an impact on professionalism. It's difficult to know where to start with taking care of yourself; however, NHS England and NHS Improvement Midlands (2020) suggest the following areas and resources:
>
> - Physical activity and diet:
>   - Active 10—a free app that supports people to walk just 10 minutes a day
>   - Couch to 5k—a free app that takes people through a programme to be able to run 5k
>   - My Fitness Pal—a free app that allows people to track food and fluid intake and physical activity
>   - Easy Meals—a free app that contains lots of simple, nutritious meals
> - Mental health: sleep and self-care:
>   - Calm—an app that offers guided meditations, sleep stories, breathing programmes and stretching exercises

Continued

TIPS—cont'd

- Sleep Life—a podcast designed to help you unlock your sleeping potential
- Thrive Mental Wellbeing—an evidence-based app to prevent and manage stress, anxiety and related conditions
- Feeling Good: positive mindset—an app that provides a programme based on positive psychology and the principles of cognitive behavioural therapy
- The Black, African and Asian Therapy Network—this website provides a list of free counselling specifically set up to serve the black and minority ethnic community
- Supporting nurses' health at work:
  - Nursing You—resources to help nurses implement changes in their work environments to better support nurses' health
- Smoking:
  - NHS Smokefree—a free app to assist you in stopping smoking with a 4-week programme of daily motivation and support
- Alcohol:
  - Drink Free Days—a free app to help you track and reduce your daily alcohol consumption by nominating drink-free days
  - Alcohol Change UK—a website that provides free resources on cutting down alcohol consumption
- Menstrual health:
  - Bloody Good Period—charity about getting sanitary pads to people who need them
  - Busting period taboos—two women who've made it their mission to smash period taboos and make it easier for girls to manage their menstrual health
  - Period Tracker—period and cycle tracker
- Menopause:
  - Manage my menopause—bespoke menopausal advice from experts in postreproductive health
  - MenoPro—an app to facilitate symptom control of menopause between doctors and women who work together

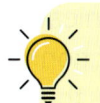

5 | NOTES ON BARRIERS AND ENABLERS TO NURSING PROFESSIONALISM

> **TIPS—cont'd**
> - Caring responsibilities:
>   - Jointly—an app that has been created for carers by carers to link carers together
>   - Carers UK Forum—an online forum where you can ask questions and access support and advice
> - Financial:
>   - Cavell—a charity that provides practical and financial support for UK nurses, midwives and healthcare assistants
>   - Money Health Check—the money advice service—free online financial health checker tool
>   - Lamplight support service—offers a telephone support service to nurses who are dealing with financial hardship
> - Hydration:
>   - Hydration Genius—a free app that allows you to log your water content to calculate the amount of water you need to stay hydrated
>   - Waterlogged Drink More Water—a free app to help you stay healthy and hydrated
> - Bereavement:
>   - Good Grief: Chat and Messaging—an app that provides you with a social network to chat, connect and grieve with others
>   - Grief Support Network—a free social networking app that allows you to connect and support people who are grieving or have grieved
>   - Bereavement and Trauma Support for our Filipino Colleagues—a confidential and free service, 7 days a week between 8 a.m. and 8 p.m.

Exhaustion

Chronic fatigue and emotional exhaustion are common among nurses, particularly in high-stress environments, affecting their cognitive functioning and emotional resilience and potentially compromising professionalism (Murray et al. 2019). Long working hours, shift work and exposure to emotionally demanding situations contribute to nurses' exhaustion, impairing their ability to communicate effectively, make sound clinical judgements and provide compassionate care. In line with the section on motivation and burnout, it is vital that nursing students get into the habit of self-care, as, ultimately, exhaustion has a potential impact on professionalism.

> **THE NMC SAYS**
>
> **20.9** Maintain the level of health you need to carry out your professional role.

Inattention to a holistic approach: Failure to adopt a holistic approach to patient care can lead to fragmented care delivery and neglect of patients' psychosocial needs, undermining nurses' professionalism and patient outcomes (Moss et al. 2017). Despite the emphasis on holistic care in nursing education and practice, time constraints, competing priorities and inadequate resources often result in a narrow focus on biomedical aspects of care, neglecting the psychological, social and spiritual dimensions of health. The effect that this can have on professionalism cannot be underestimated.

Inexperience: Transitioning into nursing student and then registered nurse can be challenging, as new graduates navigate the complexities of clinical practice, adapt to different care settings and establish their professional identity. Lack of experience may lead to feelings of insecurity, self-doubt and reluctance to assert professional autonomy, hindering nurses' ability to uphold professional standards.

ENABLERS OF NURSING PROFESSIONALISM

Just as there are barriers to nursing professionalism, there are also enablers, things that help and support nurses and nursing students in their professionalism. As with the barriers, the enablers can also be categorised into extrinsic and intrinsic; however, as with the barriers, it's essential to keep in mind that in the real world, the two are inherently linked.

Extrinsic enablers to nursing professionalism

The Nursing and Midwifery Council (NMC n.d.) suggests that the environments in which nurses and midwives work are pivotal in supporting professionalism, and it identifies five key points; these are summarised in Fig. 5.3 and expanded on as follows:

Recognition of nursing leadership

Organisations that recognise and empower nurses as leaders within interdisciplinary teams foster a culture of professionalism and facilitate nurses' engagement in decision-making processes (Cummings et al. 2018). By acknowledging nurses' expertise, leadership potential and contributions to patient care, healthcare institutions promote a sense of ownership, autonomy and accountability among nurses, enhancing their professionalism and job satisfaction. However, it goes further than the recognition of leadership: the NMC (n.d.) states that as part of that recognition of leadership, valuing the evidence-based opinion of nurses and midwives, nurses and midwives occupying roles of leadership and influence across systems, shared governance and decision making,

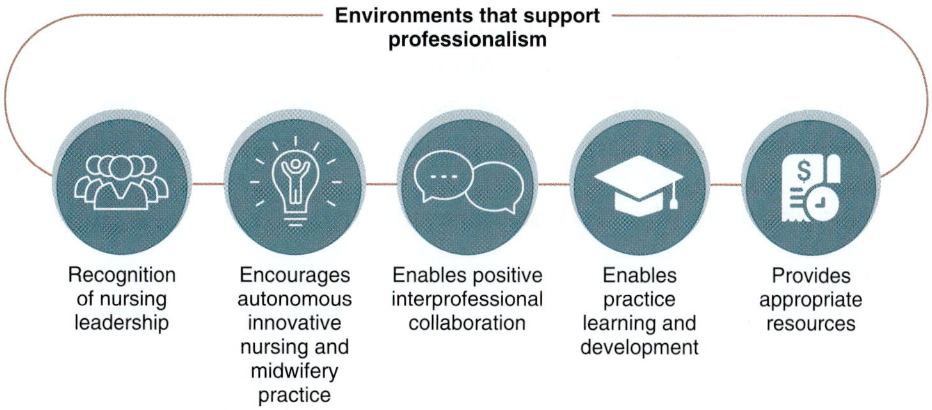

Figure 5.3 Environments that support professionalism.

and organisational risk assessment that accepts professional judgement as a basis for action also all play a role.

- Valuing the evidence-based opinion of nurses and midwives: Healthcare organisations that value and prioritise nurses' evidence-based opinions contribute to a culture of professionalism, promoting critical thinking and innovation in nursing practice (Grove et al. 2020).
- Nurses and midwives occupying roles of leadership and influence across systems: Nurses and midwives are often at the forefront of patient care delivery and possess valuable insights derived from their clinical experiences, observations and knowledge of best practices. By soliciting and incorporating nurses' perspectives into decision-making processes, organisations demonstrate respect for nurses' expertise and foster a collaborative approach to care delivery.
- Shared governance and decision making: Participation in shared governance structures empowers nurses to advocate for patient-centred care and contribute to practice development, enhancing their sense of professionalism and job satisfaction (Adamson et al. 2019). Shared governance models distribute decision-making authority across different levels of the organisation, allowing frontline nurses to have a voice in matters related to patient care standards, resource allocation and quality improvement initiatives. By involving nurses in governance processes, organisations promote transparency, accountability and professional autonomy, which are essential components of nursing professionalism.
- Organisational risk assessment that accepts professional judgement as a basis for action: As with nurses and midwives occupying roles of leadership nurses, the acceptance of professional judgement of nurses and midwives is integral, as nurses and midwives are at the forefront of patient care delivery, and they possess valuable insights.

Encouragement of autonomous and innovative practice

Encouraging autonomous and innovative practice at an organisational level can be done in a number of ways. The NMC (n.d.) recognises that the following is vital:

- Policies that support critical thinking in practice and decision making: Organisational policies that support critical thinking and

evidence-based practice enable nurses to make informed decisions and uphold professional standards in complex clinical situations (Manojlovich et al. 2019). In addition to these policies that encourage ongoing education, mentorship and interdisciplinary collaboration, they provide nurses with the necessary resources and support to critically appraise evidence, integrate research findings into practice and adapt to changing patient needs and clinical circumstances. By fostering a culture of curiosity and continuous learning, organisations empower nurses to deliver safe, effective and patient-centred care, thereby enhancing their professionalism.
- Flexibility to develop appropriate new roles—Nursing is a dynamic profession that is forever changing and evolving. Organisations that support the development of new roles are promoting nursing professionalism through respect and understanding of nursing and what nurses can do.
- Enabling practitioners to operate within the upper limits of the scope of practice: This instils pride and confidence in nurses and, indeed, nursing students, and in turn, that has an effect on professional values and professionalism.
- Providing access to expertise to support coaching and role models and practice learning—while a lack of role models is a barrier to professionalism (as identified earlier in this chapter), conversely, having access to support and role models acts as an enabler.

Encouragement of interprofessional collaboration

Collaboration with other healthcare professionals supports teamwork and enhances communication between the different levels of healthcare workers and thus improves patient care and healthcare workers', including nurses' and nursing students', satisfaction (Epstein 2014) The NMC (n.d.) suggests that interprofessional collaboration can be achieved by taking a partnership approach to team working, having clear lines of accountability and creating interprofessional learning/team-working opportunities.

> **THE NMC SAYS**
>
> 8 Work cooperatively.

> **THE NMC SAYS**
>
> **8.1** Respect the skills, expertise and contributions of your colleagues, referring matters to them when appropriate.
>
> **8.2** Maintain effective communication with colleagues.

Promotes learning and development

Provision of continuous learning opportunities and support for professional growth enhances nurses' competence and confidence, contributing to their professionalism and career satisfaction (Whitehead et al. 2018). Continuing education, certification programs and mentorship initiatives enable nurses to expand their knowledge base, refine their clinical skills and stay abreast of emerging trends and best practices in nursing. By investing in nurses' professional development, organisations demonstrate a commitment to excellence, promote retention and cultivate a culture of lifelong learning and professional growth. The NMC (n.d.) suggests this can be achieved through ensuring that preregistration programmes develop professionalism and resilience, nurses have regular supervision and a focus on reflective practice, and there is a provision of professional development opportunities and meaningful appraisal.

Provision of appropriate resources

The final area in which the NMC (n.d.) identifies extrinsic factors that can enable professionalism is around resources. Without the right resources, nurses and nursing students will find themselves in challenging circumstances where their professionalism may be tested. These resources include:

- Staffing: Earlier in the chapter, it was discussed that safe staffing can be a barrier to professionals; in contrast, getting staffing right by taking skill mix and experience into account can be an enabler to professionalism.

- Funding for learning and development: We have already mentioned the part that learning and development play in professionalism; however, without funding, this enabler cannot be realised.
- Equipment, including information technology devices and software: Having the right tools with which to provide nursing care is an essential enabler to professionalism. With the right equipment, nurses and nursing students are able to provide care with a high level of professionalism.
- Shared information and data: This, in essence, is similar to having the right equipment and another essential enabler to professionalism; again, with the right information, nurses and nursing students are able to flourish.

Intrinsic enablers to nursing professionalism

In addition to identifying extrinsic enablers to professionalism, the NMC (n.d.) also identifies intrinsic enablers to professionalism and states that "the individual practitioner is responsible for upholding his or her own professional practice". Fig. 5.4 provides an overview of how the NMC states that nurses can uphold their own professionalism.

Continuous learning and development

Nurses who prioritise continuous learning and self-improvement demonstrate a commitment to professionalism and are better equipped to adapt to evolving healthcare challenges (Brown et al. 2020). Lifelong learning is a cornerstone of nursing practice, as it enables nurses to stay current with evidence-based practices, technological advancements and regulatory changes that impact patient care delivery. By actively seeking opportunities for professional development, nurses and nursing students enhance their competence, confidence and effectiveness as healthcare providers, thereby contributing to improved patient outcomes and quality of care. The NMC (n.d.) advises that enabling professionalism through continuous learning and development can be achieved by:

- Making the most of opportunities through revalidation via existing supervision and appraisal systems: This involves nurses engaging in revalidation processes via existing supervision and appraisal

How nurses can uphold their professionalism

- Continuous learning and development
- Being a role model
- Supporting appropriate service and care environments
- Enabling person-centred care and evidence-informed practice
- Leading professionally

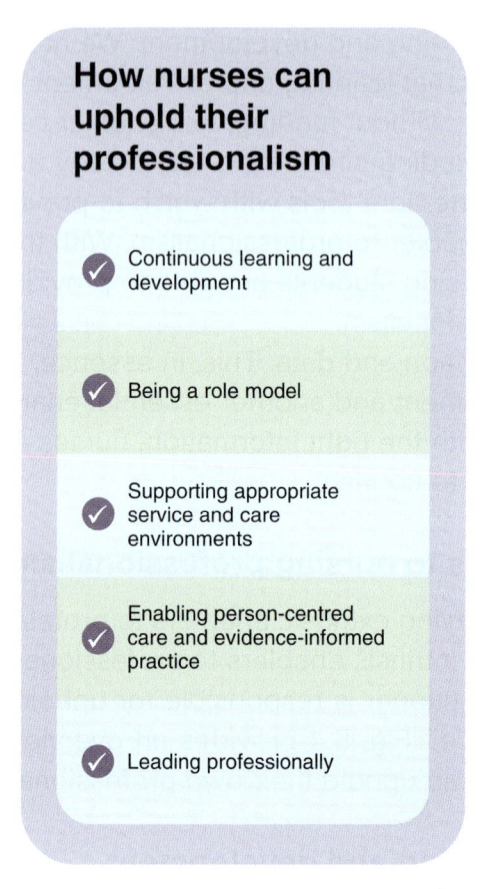

Figure 5.4 How nurses can uphold their professionalism.

systems, and it encourages nurses to reflect on their practice and identify areas for improvement, enhancing their professionalism (Wass et al. 2018). By participating in revalidation activities, nurses reaffirm their commitment to high-quality care, accountability and ongoing professional development, fostering a culture of excellence within the nursing profession.

- Accessing necessary resources to support professional development: This is about showing up, taking part, and learning and growing!
- Promoting a learning culture for others: Nurses who actively promote a learning culture within their teams facilitate the development of a supportive environment that nurtures professionalism and innovation (Rycroft-Malone et al. 2018). By fostering a culture

of continuous learning, collaboration and knowledge sharing, nurses inspire their colleagues to embrace new ideas, explore innovative practices and strive for excellence in patient care delivery. Through mentorship, coaching and peer support, nurses can create learning opportunities that empower their colleagues to develop professionally while, at the same time, growing in confidence and developing their own professionalism.

Being a role model

Nurses who exemplify professionalism and positive work attitudes serve as role models for their peers and contribute to the cultivation of a professional nursing culture (Jackson et al. 2017). Role modelling involves demonstrating ethical conduct, effective communication, clinical competence and empathy in interactions with patients, families and colleagues. By embodying the values and behaviours associated with professionalism, nurses inspire trust, confidence and respect among their peers and promote a culture of excellence and accountability within the workplace. The NMC (n.d.) identifies how nurses, nursing students, midwives and nursing associates can be role models for others, thus enabling professionalism. The first part of this is by demonstrating and articulating clearly what professionalism looks like in practice—having the ability to identify what professionalism looks and feels like is key to enabling professionalism. Tara Iles explains what professionalism looks like to her:

> 'I learned about professionalism from a young age, as both of my parents were working professionals, and my mum was a nurse. I remember being in awe of her uniform and everything it stood for. To me, it was like armour and transformed her into an important person of trust, credibility, and someone who I was very proud of. This hasn't changed, and I still view my uniform as armour, and I'm very conscious of the responsibility that comes with it, as well as my title of a registered nurse.
>
> There have been barriers to being a professional throughout my career. A large part of this has been culture. In some areas I have worked in, it

Continued

has felt relaxed and, in my opinion, not professional, to my standards anyway. By this I mean staff chewing gum, looking messy in non-ironed uniform, sitting on desks at the nurse's station or smoking outside of the hospital when wearing uniform. From a young age and as a junior member of staff, I have always felt not only incredibly sad and disheartened to view these behaviours but also embarrassed and quite irritable. I was mindful that we represent a reputable and proud profession, and members of the public viewing this will have their opinion formed very quickly, and it wouldn't be a good one. This could lead to a lack of trust for patients and/or their families and carers, and so there could in fact be real damage from nurses acting unprofessionally. We are in the privileged position of being in people's lives when they are most vulnerable, and so it is important that they trust, respect and believe us as professionals.

Some other barriers to being a professional could be ignoring problems, and this could be from personally to systematically, such as a ward or department right through to the wider picture, such as a hospital or trust. I feel strongly that the standard you walk past is the standard you accept.

Whilst it might not always be easy to respectfully challenge, we all have a duty to do so if we see something that doesn't align with our morals and values, and if it does not link to the NMC code of conduct. I have examples of challenging staff in a respectful way that hasn't always been well received. For me, I would feel more uncomfortable just walking past and ignoring it. The more senior I have become, the more I see it as part of my role to stop and question unprofessional behaviours.

It is part of my duty to understand why people might think it is acceptable and to politely explain why it is not.

Making excuses is another barrier to professionalism, and this is all too easy within healthcare. With the absolute acknowledgement that there are real issues and constraints to our healthcare system and the profession of nursing, we cannot use this as an excuse for unprofessional behaviour. We need to be careful that we don't become complacent and use 'but it was short staffed' or 'we had too many patients' when things go wrong (and they will; we don't live in a perfect world). In my many years of experience, patients, families, and carers can see and hear only too well when it might be short staffed and the pressure on the system, but it is not only our job but professional duty to make patients as safe as we can and to make them feel safe and cared for. When things do go wrong, we have a duty of candour, and to be open, honest and transparent is the only way to be. Again, my experience has taught me that this is always well received; despite the severity of the error or omission, people would always rather have the truth, and we have a professional duty to provide them with that.

Setting standards is an important part of being a professional, which I have aimed to do throughout my career. In my various roles such as a team leader to a ward sister, matron and deputy divisional director of nursing, I have been mindful that the standards I set are high, yet achievable. I have always worked to the ethos that I will never ask someone to do something that I am not prepared to do myself, and I continue to work this way. I really do think it is very important. I remember being a junior nurse and some senior nurses and sisters asking me to complete various tasks whilst they were clearly engaging in recreational conversations. I remember feeling not only undervalued but taken for granted and even mocked. I remember silently telling myself that if I ever came into a position such as theirs that I would remember that feeling and do my absolute best not to make someone else feel this way. I still work to this mantra and always will; it is part of who I am.

Some other enablers to being a professional are developing yourself constantly. We know that the NHS and healthcare is an ever-evolving system, and we need to be curious and continue to learn. To develop a professional image is important, and this will take place over time. You will build credibility with time and experience, and it has always been important to me to be a strong professional role model. I have had the luxury of having some very strong professional role models throughout

Continued

my career. They have all been very different, but the common golden thread is professionalism and appreciating their position and the fact that others can and will learn from them.

To be a true professional it is important to practice self-care. Nursing is a very physically and emotionally tolling role. In order to provide the best care for others, we have to remember to care for ourselves. This is not always easy due to our busy lives and other commitments, but it is essential to remember this. I have always encouraged staff to take their breaks, no matter how busy the shift is. I have seen all too often people saying they are too busy, which leads to resentment or even tears and burnout.

Personally, I have, and always will pride myself on my professionalism, but I balance that with humility and compassion. I don't ever want to be a robot who just speaks of policies and buzzwords. Actions are louder than words, and I think building connections with people and allowing them to see you in practice is powerful. Integrity, compassion, and professionalism are some of the traits that I remain most proud of'.

Tara Iles, RN, BSc (Hons), MSc, MSc (distinction), senior nurse, Women's Health Quality, Sustainability and Innovation, Nursing Directorate, NHS England

What does professionalism look like to you? Can you articulate it clearly so that others can understand?

_____
_____
_____
_____
_____
_____

5 | NOTES ON BARRIERS AND ENABLERS TO NURSING PROFESSIONALISM

Another intrinsic enabler that the NMC (n.d.) identifies in relation to being a role model is that nurses and nursing students should demonstrate positive behaviours and attitudes towards diversity. Nurses who demonstrate respect for diversity and inclusivity contribute to a culturally competent healthcare environment and uphold professional values of equity and justice (Crenshaw et al., 2020). In today's increasingly diverse society, nursing students will encounter patients from various cultural, ethnic and socioeconomic backgrounds, each with unique healthcare needs and preferences. By embracing diversity and fostering cultural competence, nursing students and, indeed, nurses can create a welcoming and inclusive care environment that promotes trust, engagement and collaboration among patients, families and healthcare providers. This, in turn, has an impact on enabling and supporting professionalism at all levels.

> **THE NMC SAYS**
>
> **1.3** Avoid making assumptions and recognise diversity and individual choice.

Other ways in which the NMC (n.d.) suggests that nursing professionalism can be enabled through being a role model is by:

- Working within a clear professional career framework
- Supporting colleagues and students
- Celebrating personal success and that of others
- Developing people to take on senior roles and supporting those in senior roles
- Treating others with a positive regard
- Providing meaningful and constructive feedback to others

Enabling person-centred and evidence-led practice

- Incorporating up-to-date evidence in daily practice
- Sharing and disseminating evidence-informed practice
- Participation in the generation of new evidence and working innovatively
- Lobbying for change and improvement

Being a professional leader

Leadership has been a common theme throughout the enablers section of this chapter. Mrayyan et al (2023) states, 'Engaging in clinical leadership is an obligation, not a choice, for all clinicians at all levels. This obligation is more critical in nursing with many emerging global health issues, such as the COVID-19 pandemic'. And this is echoed in the NMC code:

> **THE NMC SAYS**
>
> **25** Provide leadership to make sure people's well-being is protected and to improve their experiences of the health and care system.

The NMC (n.d.) suggests that nurses and nursing students can enable professionalism through leadership by:

- Seeking connection to and support from professional bodies and organisations
- Developing self to lead strategically
- Developing others to lead strategically
- Supporting those in leadership

Supporting appropriate care environments

It seems appropriate to come full circle within this chapter, which started with exploring the barrier to professionalism that care environments can be. To complete the circle, we now look at care environments within the context of them being intrinsic enablers of professionalism and how nurses and nursing students can support appropriately. The NMC (n.d.) states that this can be achieved through:

- Raising concerns when issues arise that could compromise safety, quality and experience
- Supporting others to raise concerns appropriately
- Defining and understanding clear referral pathways to support standards of professional practice
- Delegate tasks and duties safely
- Identifying appropriate professional support networks for self and others
- Working collegiately with other professions

5 | NOTES ON BARRIERS AND ENABLERS TO NURSING PROFESSIONALISM

CONCLUSION

In conclusion, nursing professionalism is influenced by a myriad of factors, both intrinsic and extrinsic, that shape nurses' attitudes, behaviours and practices. While barriers such as challenging care environments, lack of role models and burnout can impede nurses' ability to exhibit professionalism, enablers such as recognition of nursing leadership, valuing evidence-based practice and professional development opportunities can enhance their professional practice and contribute to positive patient outcomes. By addressing these barriers and leveraging enablers, nursing students can support and help to create a supportive environment conducive to nursing professionalism, ultimately improving patient safety, quality of care and overall healthcare outcomes.

Space for reader's own reflection:

REFERENCES

Adamson, K.A., Bumbak, L.M., Daulton, B.J., 2019. Shared governance and nurse empowerment: The influence on nursing-sensitive patient outcomes. J. Nurs. Manag 27 (1), 91–97.

Babaei, S., Taleghani, F., 2019. Compassionate Care Challenges and Barriers in Clinical Nurses: A Qualitative Study. Iran J. Nurs. Midwifery Res 24 (3), 213–219.

Brown, J., Aitken, L.M., Marshall, A.P., 2020. Barriers and facilitators to nurses' participation in continuing education in a regional acute care hospital: An integrative review. J. Contin. Educ. Nurs 51 (1), 27–34.

Chapman, R., Rahman, A., Courtney, M., Chalmers, C., 2018. Nursing characteristics and the work environment in psychiatric inpatient units. Issues Ment. Health Nurs 39 (3), 231–238.

Crenshaw, K., Sievers, A., Williams, J., 2020. Advancing diversity and inclusion in nursing education: The Mississippi perspective. J. Nurs. Educ 59 (8), 437–440.

Cummings, G.G., Tate, K., Lee, S., Wong, C.A., Paananen, T., 2018. Leadership styles and outcome patterns for the nursing workforce and work environment: A systematic review. Int. J. Nurs. Stud 85, 19–60.

Dall'Ora, C., Saville, C., 2021. Burnout in nursing: What have we learnt and what is still unknown? Nurs. Times [online], 117 (2), 43–44.

Elliott, M., Coventry, L., 2020. Can compassion be learned? A mixed methods longitudinal design addressing empathy and attitude in undergraduate nursing education. Nurse Educ. Today 92, 123–129.

Epstein, N.E., 2014. Multidisciplinary in-hospital teams improve patient outcomes: A review. Surg. Neurol. Int 5 (Suppl 7), S295–S303.

Griffiths, P., Maruotti, A., Recio-Saucedo, A., Redfern, O. C., 2018. Nurse staffing, nursing assistants and hospital mortality: Retrospective longitudinal cohort study. BMJ Qual. Saf 27 (10), 832–840.

Grove, S.K., Burns, N., Gray, J., 2020. The practice of nursing research: Appraisal, synthesis, and generation of evidence, ninth ed. Elsevier.

Health and Care Professions Council. 2014. Professionalism in healthcare professionals [Online]. https://www.hcpc-uk.org/globalassets/resources/reports/professionalism-in-healthcare-professionals.pdf [Accessed April 15, 2024]

Hutchinson, M., Jackson, D., 2019. Hostile clinician behaviours in the nursing work environment and implications for patient care: A mixed-methods systematic review. BMC Nurs 18 (1), 53.

Hupcey, J.E., Penrod, J., Morse, J.M., Mitcham, C., 2018. An exploration and advancement of the concept of trust. J. Adv. Nurs 74 (3), 580–591.

Jackson, D., Andrew, S., Cleary, M., Walter, G., 2017. Understanding burnout in nursing: A literature review. J. Nurs. Manag 25 (5), 406–415.

Jackson, D., Firtko, A., Edenborough, M., 2020. Personal resilience as a strategy for surviving and thriving in the face of workplace adversity: A literature review. J. Adv. Nurs 72 (9), 2002–2015.

Manojlovich, M., Laschinger, H.K.S., Kerr, M.S., 2019. Staff nurse empowerment and effort-reward imbalance. J. Nurs. Manag 27 (6), 1271–1280.

Morrison, D., 2021. Vivid Method. Transcript: The standard you walk past is the standard you accept [Online]. https://vividmethod.com/transcript-the-standard-you-walk-past-is-the-standard-you-accept/ [Accessed April 15, 2024]

Moss, K.O., Taylor, D., Hoffart, N., 2017. Holistic nursing care: A requirement for quality care? Br. J. Nurs 26 (22), 1256–1261.

Mrayyan, M.T, Algunmeeyn, A., Abunab, H.Y., et al, 2023. Attributes, skills and actions of clinical leadership in nursing as reported by hospital nurses: a cross-sectional study. BMJ Leader 2023, 7, 203–211.

Murray, M., Sundin, D., Cope, V., 2019. Challenges and opportunities in nursing documentation: Perceptions of nurses working on the frontline of care. J. Clin. Nurs 28 (13–14), 2450–2458.

NHS England and NHS Improvement Midlands. 2020. Caring for Yourself: A guide for frontline NHS staff [Online]. https://www.england.nhs.uk/midlands/wp-content/uploads/sites/46/2020/10/NHS_Caring_for_Yourself_FINAL_MIDLANDS_201002.pdf [Accessed April 15, 2024]

Nursing and Midwifery Council. n.d. Enabling Professionalism [Online]. https://www.nmc.org.uk/globalassets/sitedocuments/other-publications/enabling-professionalism.pdfhttps://www.nmc.org.uk/globalassets/sitedocuments/other-publications/enabling-professionalism.pdf [Accessed April 16, 2024]

Rycroft-Malone, J., Seers, K., Chandler, J., Hawkes, C.A., Crichton, N., Allen, C., Bullock, I., & Strunin, L., 2018. The role of evidence, context, and facilitation in an implementation trial: Implications for the development of the PARIHS framework. Implement. Sci 13 (1), 1–13.

Sharp, S., Mcallister, M., Broadbent, M., 2018. The tension between person centred care and task focused care in an acute surgical setting: A critical ethnography. Collegian 25, (1), 11–17.

Terry, L.M., Carr, G.J., Curzio, J., 2019. Older adults' experiences of receiving care from undergraduate student nurses: A systematic review of qualitative studies. Int. J. Nurs. Stud 92, 109–120.

Wass, V., Van der Vleuten, C., Shatzer, J., Jones, R., 2018. Assessment of clinical competence. Lancet 389 (10066), 197–198.

Whitehead, P.B., Herbertson, R.K., Hamric, A.B., Epstein, E.G., Fisher, J.M., 2018. Moral distress among healthcare professionals: Report of an institution-wide survey. J. Nurs Sch 50 (6), 636–644.

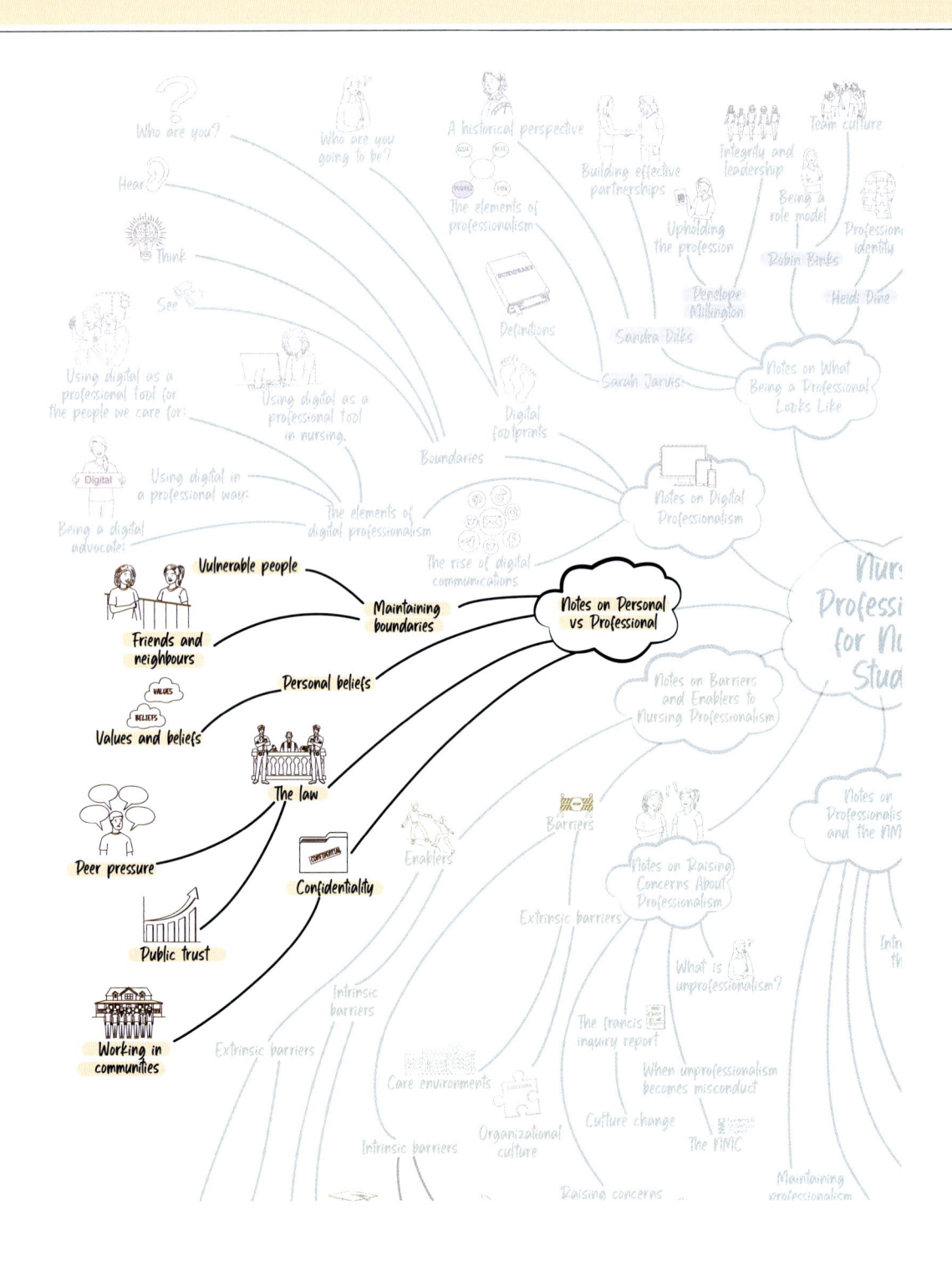

Notes on Personal vs Professional

- Maintaining boundaries
  - Vulnerable people
  - Friends and neighbours
- Personal beliefs
  - Values and beliefs
- The law
  - Peer pressure
  - Public trust
- Confidentiality
  - Working in communities

6

NOTES ON PERSONAL VERSUS PROFESSIONAL

Hayley Jones (she/her)

INTRODUCTION

Nursing values, as set out by the Nursing and Midwifery Council (NMC), 'The code: Professional standards of practice and behaviours for nurses, midwives and nursing associates' (2018), apply both in and out of the workplace. How nurses conduct themselves in and out of work can lead to personal and professional dilemmas. Nursing students need to grasp the need to consider how we portray ourselves to colleagues, the patients we care for and the communities in which we live from the very beginning. Every nurse has a right to a personal life that is private and separate from our working life, but there are times when our behaviours or the actions that we take cross over from our personal to our professional lives (or vice versa). The impact of these behaviours and/or actions can be against what is expected of us professionally in line with the code and can, at times, have serious consequences. This chapter will consider some of these scenarios and the potential personal and/or professional dilemmas we can be faced with as a result.

WHAT IS MEANT BY THE TERM 'PROFESSION'?

The term profession refers to a job role that requires a high level of education and training and is recognised by the general public as a group of individuals with a specialist set of skills. Nursing falls into this category, as all nursing students are required to be educated to degree level as a minimum standard to be entered into the register as a registered nurse.

> 'What does profession mean to me? It means a sense of belonging. Belonging to a group of individuals that are proud of what they do. Profession to me means an identity that goes beyond a uniform. It is conduct, it is standards, it is competence, it is training, it is recognition and it is a sense of duty'.
>
> **Bethan Williams, registered nurse**

> 'A profession means having integrity. It is about being trustworthy and doing the right thing regardless of personal feelings or opinions. It is more than a job, it is who you are and all that goes with it'.
>
> **Lisa Morris, MSc, registered nurse**

The professionalisation of nurses has occurred over many years through education and innovation and has proven to be the focus of significant and ongoing discussions. Across the world, nurses have developed themselves into professionals with a great deal of knowledge (Hoeve et al. 2014). Ghadirian et al. (2014) explore the evolution of nursing as a profession, stating that for many years, nursing was seen as a semiprofession due to the lack of academics at the entry level and the lack of theory and theory-based research. However, with the development of educational standards and strong connections between nursing and research, this has changed significantly, with the Royal College of Nursing (2024) defining nursing as 'a safety critical profession founded on four pillars: clinical practice, education, research, and leadership. Registered nurses use evidence-based knowledge, professional and clinical judgement to assess, plan, implement and evaluate high-quality person-centred nursing care'.

WHY ARE NURSING PROFESSIONAL STANDARDS IMPORTANT?

The NMC is the governing body for nurses, midwives and nursing associates. The NMC (2023) states that its core role is to regulate, and it does this through promoting high education and professional standards for nurses and midwives across the United Kingdom and nursing associates in England. The NMC also maintains the register of professionals eligible to practise and investigate concerns about nurses, midwives and nursing associates. The NMC has a responsibility to the public to ensure that, as a profession, we follow a set of professional standards, a set of values, behaviours and principles that the general public expects of us as healthcare professionals. When we register as a nurse with the relevant qualifications (and subsequent reregistrations), we agree to follow these values, behaviours and principles. If these are not followed, action can be taken by the NMC, and in some cases, the nurse can be removed from the register. In the United Kingdom, nobody can practise as a registered nurse without being on the NMC register.

There are four sections to the Code:

1. Prioritise people
2. Practise effectively
3. Preserve safety
4. Promote professionalism and trust

> **THE NMC SAYS**
>
> **Promote professionalism and trust**
>
> You uphold the reputation of your profession at all times. You should display a personal commitment to the standards of practice and behaviour set out in the Code. You should be a model of integrity and leadership for others to aspire to. This should lead to trust and confidence in the professions from patients, people receiving care, other health and care professionals and the public.
>
> **20.** Uphold the reputation of your profession at all times.
>
> **20.1** Keep to and uphold the standards and values set out in the code.

PROFESSIONAL AND PERSONAL DILEMMAS IN NURSING

As a working registered nurse and a nursing student, the likelihood is that you deliver nursing care to members of the community within the area in which you live. At some point, this nursing care will be to people we know who live locally, close friends and/or relatives we know personally. How we behave in and out of the work environment is important at all times once we are registrants. If you do not follow the values, behaviours and principles of our profession outside of work as well as during your working day, you can bring your profession into disrepute, meaning you can damage the overall reputation of all nurses.

As humans, we have a tendency to remember negative experiences far more easily than we remember the positive ones, and for the general public, this is very true.

SOCIAL MEDIA X
@silverangel882

It's (professionalism) about being the best nurse I can be and following the code to support that. But also being a role model in both my professional life and private life. But in todays age of social media our behaviours can be shared instantly and any errors of judgement are immortalised.

Think about some of the poor publicity nurses have had in the press as a result of poor behaviour by just one registered nurse. How do you think this has affected the overall reputation of nurses? Do you think opinions about what we do as nurses changes when the profession receives poor publicity?

6 | NOTES ON PERSONAL VERSUS PROFESSIONAL

_____
_____
_____
_____
_____
_____

For some people who know very little about the nursing profession, opinions are formed through hearsay, listening to the experience of others they know, listening to the news and reading papers and social media. While nursing continues to be the most trusted profession, with 89% of British people trusting nurses to tell the truth and just 12% trusting politicians (putting them in last place) (Royal College of Nursing 2022), the public's perception of nursing as a profession is diverse and muddled. The general public has little comprehension of the many areas of nursing work, and there is a disparity between what nurses actually do and what the public perceives they do (Blau et al. 2023). The public's understanding of nursing generally comes from the media or is rooted in long-standing myths and stories of angels carrying lamps and mopping brows. It's important to realise this disparity and remember that, depending on the nature of the story being told or the incident being reported, any inaccuracies or biased views could potentially give the receiver of that information a different perception. With your insight, though, you, as a future registered nurse, may have a different understanding. In these circumstances, confidentiality, policies and procedures are really important, and so, we often find ourselves unable to correct misinformation, as we could be breaking confidentiality, policies and procedures that are in place to safeguard our patients, ourselves and colleagues. This can present a dilemma, particularly about an experience, subject or situation you feel very strongly about, as you are unable to talk about the events as you understand them.

The next few sections explore some personal/professional dilemmas. Of course, these are not all of the personal/professional dilemmas you may encounter as a nurse; however, the case studies may help you, as a nursing student, to recognise and think through dilemmas when you encounter them. All of the case studies are fictional; however, all are possible.

PERSONAL/PROFESSIONAL DILEMMA: CONFIDENTIALITY

One of the most challenging dilemmas can be maintaining confidentiality because, as nurses, we are often part of the communities we work in.

> **NMC**
>
> **THE NMC SAYS**
>
> **5** Respect people's right to privacy and confidentiality.
>
> As a nurse, midwife or nursing associate, you owe a duty of confidentiality to all those who are receiving care. This includes making sure that they are informed about their care and that information about them is shared appropriately.

Confidentiality, on the surface, seems like an easy win. In simple terms, it's about not disclosing information about the people we care for to people who are not part of that care in one way or another. However, this can feel more challenging when we come into contact with someone we know. For example, a close friend has a relative you are caring for; in this situation, you need to be very careful who you share information with and the level of information that is shared. We live in a complex society where family dynamics and social relationships can be difficult at best. To assume a patient is happy for their information to be shared with any family member and then doing so can lead to serious consequences for you as a registrant. We can all find ourselves in situations where we may share information without thinking of the consequences,

6 | NOTES ON PERSONAL VERSUS PROFESSIONAL

particularly if we are among friends and family, and it's this type of dynamic that leads to personal and professional dilemmas. The case study that follows illustrates this point.

CASE STUDY

Annabelle is a registered nurse who works in a local community hospital on a ward with elderly patients who require further rehabilitation and/or further assessment for ongoing care needs. Annabelle lives locally and is often caring for relatives of her friends in her local community. On one occasion, Annabelle is caring for an elderly gentleman who has the capacity to make decisions for himself. He is the uncle of an old school friend she knows well. Annabelle has not seen the old school friend for some time and bumps into her on a night out during her time off. The relative of the elderly gentleman starts chatting to Annabelle, and after a few alcoholic drinks, the old school friend mentions to Annabelle that her uncle is in hospital and she is very concerned about him. Without thinking, Annabelle replies that she knows her uncle and has been caring for him, and she seeks to reassure her old school friend that he is, in fact, doing well. The school friend proceeds to question Annabelle in a way that would make Annabelle think they have a close relationship, as she divulges some personal information about her uncle's ongoing care needs.

Following the night out Annabelle had with her friends, her old school friend relays the personal information about her uncle's ongoing care needs to another member of the family. It transpires that the family had a big falling out over an inheritance the uncle received that was disputed by the rest of the family, and they no longer communicate. However, the ongoing care needs means he will have to use the inheritance to help pay for his ongoing care, and the family is outraged, as they have yet to settle the matter in the courts. Family members arrived on the ward, and arguments between the family members became very unpleasant. The police were called to help remove the family members from the ward, as they refused to leave. The ward manager undertakes an investigation, and the breach of

Continued

> **CASE STUDY—cont'd**
>
> confidentiality is identified. Annabelle is asked for a formal statement, after which a disciplinary hearing is held, and Annabelle is given a final written warning lasting for 12 months for breaching confidentiality outside of the workplace.

This was a very serious lesson for Annabelle. Annabelle breached this patient's confidentiality. Partly, this was due to alcohol and the fact that alcohol lowers inhibitions, meaning we are more likely to say or do something we would usually stop ourselves from doing if we were sober. However, partly, this could have been due to Annabelle not taking a moment to consider and recognise this as a personal/professional dilemma.

> **TIPS**
>
> Tips on maintaining confidentiality in social situations:
>
> Maintain boundaries and be clear to friends and family: Your friends and family need to understand that you cannot talk about the care you deliver to their relatives or close friends, and be clear they should not be asking you.
>
> Be polite but firm: If friends or family push for information, being clear that you cannot divulge any information will reduce the risk of further questions being asked of you.
>
> Refer to the NMC code: It's a good idea to explain to friends and family about the NMC code of conduct and what this means for you and your role.
>
> Be mindful: There is no rule or part of the NMC code that states nurses cannot drink alcohol, but be mindful that if you are caring for someone that you are connected with socially, alcohol can lower inhibitions and lead to sticky situations.
>
> Discuss the situation with a colleague: Remember you are never alone; pick up the phone, and talk to a trusted colleague about the situation.

6 | NOTES ON PERSONAL VERSUS PROFESSIONAL

> **TIPS—cont'd**
>
> **Be honest:** If you do find yourself in any situation where confidentiality has been breached, then be honest, talk to your manager and explain what has happened.

PERSONAL/PROFESSIONAL DILEMMA: THE LAW

The NMC code is very succinct but very clear when it comes to the law.

> **THE NMC SAYS**
>
> **20.4** Keep to the laws of the country in which you are practising.

The NMC (2024) also states, 'Sometimes the way a nurse, midwife or nursing associate conducts themselves outside their professional practice can be serious professional misconduct and will require us to act. We will take action when a professional's conduct:

- either indicates deep-seated attitudinal issues which could pose a risk to the public in professional practice, or
- is capable of undermining public trust and confidence in the profession, raising fundamental questions about the nurse, midwife or nursing associate's ability to uphold the values and standards set out in the Code'.

Following on from the case study earlier in this chapter involving Annabelle, the next personal/professional dilemma case study looks at a different type of social situation and the use of recreational drugs—drugs that are taken for enjoyment and are typically illegal. For some people, taking recreational drugs is preferred over drinking alcohol, and sometimes they will take a combination of the two. The Crown Prosecution Service (n.d.) states, 'It is illegal to possess, supply and produce controlled drugs', and 'carrying controlled drugs is illegal and you can be charged even if you did not know what you had was a controlled drug or if the drugs are yours or not'. Nurses and nursing students who find themselves in social situations where friends take recreational drugs in their presence face a huge personal/professional dilemma, and it is important that they realise the potential professional impact. This can be a really difficult situation to manage. The case study that follows explores a dilemma involving recreational drugs.

> **CASE STUDY**
>
> Harry is a newly qualified registered nurse who works on a medical ward in a hospital. During a night out with friends, after having a few alcoholic drinks, Harry is encouraged by his friend to take a pill—it is a recreational drug. Harry is unsure and feels nervous about the situation, so he takes a moment to step outside and get some fresh air and to consider what to do. Harry is aware of the NMC code of conduct and what it states about the law. Harry decides that he will not take the recreational drug and tells his friends of his decision. A short while later, there is an altercation between one of Harry's friends and another person. The police are called and intervene. The police suspect that some members of the group have taken recreational drugs, and a search of each person present is carried out. The police are happy that Harry is not involved and he has no recreational drugs, so they do not take any further action.
>
> The next day, Harry reflects on the situation and decides to phone a close colleague, who is a more experienced registered nurse, to discuss what happened. Harry's colleague listens to Harry, and they talk about personal/professional dilemmas and the NMC code. They reflect on the potential impact that recreational drug use could have on Harry and even the people Harry cares for. Harry's colleague tells Harry that it was a difficult situation that he found himself in, but ultimately, he made the right decision.

To make a professional decision in a social situation is a difficult task. The case study involving Harry was simplistic, but in reality, there could have been many factors at play: peer pressure, alcohol, friendship, confidence, experience, environment and so much more. What Harry was able to do was recognise that this was a personal/professional dilemma and step outside to reflect on what was happening. Had Harry taken or been in possession of recreational drugs and been arrested, he could have received a police caution (or more). In this situation, Harry would have had no option but to inform his line manager and the NMC. This would have resulted in a disciplinary investigation and a subsequent hearing. Ultimately, Harry would have been risking his registration with the NMC and his role as a registered nurse.

> What do you think about the repercussions? Is taking illicit drugs worth the risk of losing your job? Or having to disclose it every time you apply for a new post and potentially being removed from the NMC register? How do you think future employers might view you when shortlisting for posts or considering you for a promotion?
>
> _____
> _____
> _____
> _____
> _____
> _____

PERSONAL/PROFESSIONAL DILEMMA: PERSONAL BELIEFS

Ethical dilemmas are something that nurses and nursing students face as part of their daily practice. In one study by Raines (2000), it was found that oncology nurses alone experienced an average of 32 ethical dilemmas over a year during their day-to-day practice. Ethical dilemmas are defined as 'a situation in which a difficult choice has to be made between two courses of action, either of which entails transgressing a moral principle' (Oxford Languages 2024) Personal beliefs can lead to ethical dilemmas for nurses and nursing students. The NMC code provides some guidance on this.

> **THE NMC SAYS**
>
> **20.2** Act with honesty and integrity at all times, treating people fairly and without discrimination, bullying or harassment.
>
> **20.7** Make sure you do not express your personal beliefs (including political, religious or moral beliefs) to people in an inappropriate way.

We all have our individual values and beliefs. Some things, we can feel quite strongly about. Some things go against our moral code, but as registered nurses, every patient we care for has a right to the same standard of high-quality care as the next person, no matter what they may have done in the past, what they continue to do or what they believe in.

> **SOCIAL MEDIA X**
> **@RakheeLb**
>
> Nurse-patient relationship is essential. Effective communication, information sharing. Build trust & respect enable both parties to feel safe & able to build a good therapeutic relationship. Empathy, advocating for the patient, providing feedback.

> **SOCIAL MEDIA X**
> **@Bartonrd Confession**
>
> I have cared for patients I did not like. The personal & professional challenge was to reflect on my own behaviour.

Our own values, beliefs, likes and dislikes can be very difficult to manage. It can become even more difficult if you are made aware of something someone has done that goes against everything you believe in. The following case study explores one registered nurse's personal belief and how this created a personal/professional dilemma.

> **CASE STUDY**
> Sarah is a registered nurse who works in the emergency department. Sarah has had several miscarriages over the past few years and is yet to carry a baby to full term. She is having a difficult time coming to terms with this and is desperate to be a mum. During a weekend night shift, Sarah admits a teenage girl who has attempted to abort her unborn child herself; she is 5 months pregnant. She admits to knowing for some time but thought if she ignored it long enough, it would go away. She was unsuccessful but is crying constantly that she needs to 'get rid of it' and begs Sarah not to call her parents, as she fears their reaction if they find out she is pregnant. Sarah is really struggling with providing the standard of care this young girl needs.

This is just one example where an individual, the registered nurse, is struggling with a personal issue and then professionally is faced with having to care for a patient, which highlights that personal issue in their professional world. A different example could include having to provide nursing care to a patient who has just carried out an act of terrorism where dozens of people have been injured or, worse, died, and you have to provide nursing care to the same standard as those who have been injured. Or a person who is a convicted paedophile is admitted to your ward or service, and all you can think about are your own children, your nieces and nephews, and friends' children. The list is endless. During your nursing career, you will, no doubt, face situations where you feel you cannot deliver a high standard of care to someone who has done something you do not agree with. So how do you manage this? How do you ensure the patient does receive the standard of care they are entitled to? How do you ensure you follow the NMC code?

Thinking about the case study given here. How can Sarah ensure the teenage girl has the care she needs?

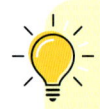

_____
_____
_____
_____
_____
_____

TIPS

Remember that you are not alone but part of a team. If you find yourself having to care for someone and this is personally challenging for you, talk about it with your manager, your university or a trusted colleague. Reflect on your feelings and what support you may need. Ask for help if you need it.

During your nursing training, you may find that your values and beliefs are challenged. This can be confusing and unsettling as you really start to think about why you think and feel the way you do about a variety of issues. You may question why your thoughts and feelings about certain issues are being challenged in this way. Please be assured that it is to ensure you are clear in your own mind why you think and feel the way you do. This, in turn, can help you identify the group of patients to whom you may struggle to deliver a high standard of care. What you do about it is just as important.

PERSONAL/PROFESSIONAL DILEMMA: MAINTAINING BOUNDARIES

There may be times where you are allocated the care of a patient you know particularly well. How do you think that would make you feel? Would it be the right thing to do—provide care for someone you know well? It all depends on the circumstances.

> **THE NMC SAYS**
>
> **20.6** Stay objective and have clear professional boundaries at all times with people in your care (including those who have been in your care in the past), their families and carers.

Depending on your nursing role and the level of care you are providing, it may be that you can deliver care to someone you know very well. An example might be someone who works in the minor injuries unit and is treating their neighbour for an injury they have sustained at home. As long as a professional exchange is maintained and it does not become personal, it could be considered appropriate for you to deliver that care. However, if the setting was an inpatient ward and you were having to provide personal care that included assisting with bathing or washing, you and your neighbour might feel more uncomfortable. After all, you may feel awkward seeing your neighbour once they have been discharged from hospital if you have had to support them with personal care of an intimate nature. In these circumstances, in order to maintain the professional boundary, you would need to raise your concerns with your team manager and ask for the patient to be reallocated to another colleague.

> Think about how you would manage a situation that involved a close family member being admitted to your ward for specialist care. If there was no alternative suitable environment for them to be admitted to, what would you do?
>
> _____
>
> _____
>
> _____
>
> _____
>
> _____
>
> _____

If a close family member were to be admitted to your place of work, the best course of action would be to have a discussion with your team manager. It would not be appropriate for you to deliver care to your family member while you are working. You may be in a position to ensure you work on the opposite side of the ward; you may be able to ensure you are not assigned to the visit if you work in the community setting, or you may wish to think about asking to be moved to another area on a temporary basis while your family member is being cared for in your working environment. Bed managers will consider where the most appropriate ward is for the needs of the patient; if there is a clear conflict of interest, it may be worth a discussion to ask if there is another area that can carry out the required specialist care.

Maintaining professional boundaries also extends to developing new relationships. Imagine you are working, you are single and you meet a patient with whom there is a mutual attraction.

6 | NOTES ON PERSONAL VERSUS PROFESSIONAL

THE NMC SAYS

20.2 Act with honesty and integrity at all times, treating people fairly and without discrimination, bullying or harassment.

20.5 Treat people in a way that does not take advantage of their vulnerability or cause them upset or distress.

20.6 Stay objective and have clear professional boundaries at all times with people in your care (including those who have been in your care in the past), their families and carers.

Applying the points of the code outlined here, acting with honesty and integrity, not taking advantage of someone's vulnerability and having clear professional boundaries, you should not allow any kind of relationship to develop with a patient before or after their episode of care has finished.

> What would you do? Do you think that sounds harsh? Not being able to start a relationship even after the patient has been discharged from your care?
>
> _____
> _____
> _____
> _____
> _____
> _____

Patients undergoing an episode of care are often in a vulnerable position; they could be unwell or have a condition that needs nursing input. It is easy for patients to develop feelings they may not under normal circumstances. They see you from a different perspective. People can often describe nurses as 'angels' or 'saviours', particularly if their condition was life threatening. They watch you working hard, caring for patients with a warm and nurturing demeanour. They are 'wowed' by your ability to carry out a number of tasks while still calming the elderly, confused patient who continues to try and escape the ward. You ask for personal information; you want to know what matters to them and what their worries are while they are in hospital. But you must remember they are in a vulnerable position. They are under your care, and to start a relationship before or after an episode of care has finished is considered ethically wrong.

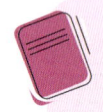

> **CASE STUDY**
> Louise is a mental health nurse in an inpatient mental health hospital. She meets John, who has been admitted after trying to take his own life and is diagnosed with severe depression for which he needs assessment, medication and ongoing review. During a prolonged stay of 3 months, while they try to get the dose of medication right and support John to get home again, Louise and John have got to know each other well. Part of Louise's role as a mental health nurse is to try and understand what worries John and what makes him 'tick' so they can tailor aspects of his care to meet his needs. John feels attracted to Louise; he thinks she is very pretty, and he thinks she is genuinely interested in him. During their discussions, it becomes apparent that they have many of the same interests. Louise is conscious that professional boundaries are at risk of being blurred.

Remshardt (2012) states that 'by virtue of our profession, there are many situations in which our designated boundaries allow for intimate entry into another person's life experiences'. However, embarking on a personal relationship with a patient, past or present, can put your NMC registration and your contract of employment at risk. In addition to this, as a coworker, if you become aware of an inappropriate relationship, you have a professional responsibility to report it. Griffith (2013) states, 'The NMC is clear, the relationship between nurses and patients is a

6 | NOTES ON PERSONAL VERSUS PROFESSIONAL

therapeutic caring relationship. It can never be about building personal or social contacts and to do so is regarded as an abuse of power and professional misconduct'. Griffith (2013) goes on to outline breaches of professional boundaries between a nurse and a patient and behaviours indicative of a move towards a breach. Fig. 6.1 depicts these points.

Breaches of professional boundaries between a nurse and a patient
- Starting a personal relationship during or after treatment
- Engaging in sexual activity with a patient
- Discussions involving sexual matters that are not relevant to treatment
- The use of sexual humour or telling 'dirty jokes'
- Engaging repeatedly in prolonged conversation about personal matters unrelated to treatment
- Criminal sexual activity

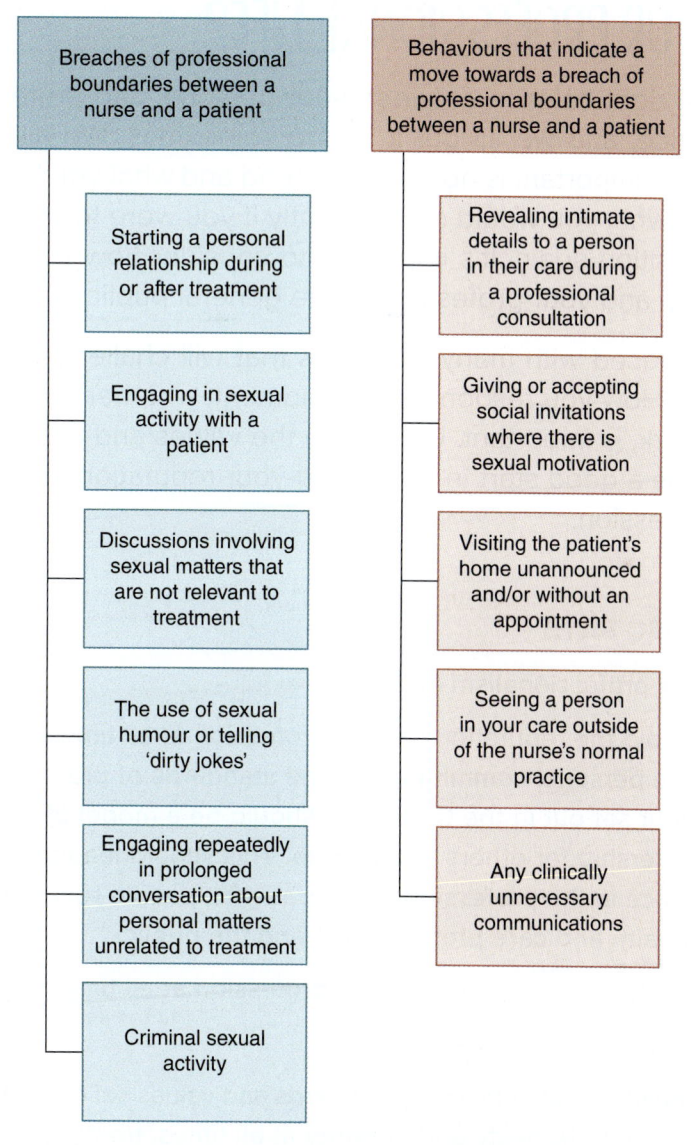

Behaviours that indicate a move towards a breach of professional boundaries between a nurse and a patient
- Revealing intimate details to a person in their care during a professional consultation
- Giving or accepting social invitations where there is sexual motivation
- Visiting the patient's home unannounced and/or without an appointment
- Seeing a person in your care outside of the nurse's normal practice
- Any clinically unnecessary communications

Figure 6.1   Professional boundarie.

For Louise, the registered nurse in the case study, the course of action is clear; she is unable to pursue a relationship with John, and if she does, she puts her NMC registration at risk.

HOW DO WE BALANCE OUR PERSONAL LIFE WITH OUR PROFESSIONAL LIFE?

Getting the right balance between your personal and professional life takes practice, and we all get it wrong sometimes. We all make mistakes; what is important is how you respond and what you learn, and be clear about what you would do differently if you were to find yourself in a similar position again. It's important to consider how your behaviour portrays you and your profession to the general public.

You will be faced with many situations that will challenge your values and beliefs. How you respond in the moment, whether you are in work or out of work, is important. Upholding the values and principles of the NMC code is a good start in protecting your reputation and that of the nursing profession.

> **THE NMC SAYS**
>
> **Promote professionalism and trust**
>
> You uphold the reputation of your profession at all times. You should display a personal commitment to the standards of practice and behaviour set out in the Code. You should be a model of integrity and leadership for others to aspire to. This should lead to trust and confidence in the professions from patients, people receiving care, other health and care professionals and the public.
>
> **20.** Uphold the reputation of your profession at all times
>
> To achieve this, you must:
>
> 20.1 Keep to and uphold the standards and values set out in the Code.
> 20.2 Act with honesty and integrity at all times, treating people fairly and without discrimination, bullying or harassment.

NMC

20.3 Be aware at all times of how your behaviour can affect and influence the behaviour of other people.

20.4 Keep to the laws of the country in which you are practising.

20.5 Treat people in a way that does not take advantage of their vulnerability or cause them upset or distress.

20.6 Stay objective and have clear professional boundaries at all times with people in your care (including those who have been in your care in the past), their families and carers.

20.7 Make sure you do not express your personal beliefs (including political, religious or moral beliefs) to people in an inappropriate way.

20.8 Act as a role model of professional behaviour for students and newly qualified nurses, midwives and nursing associates to aspire to.

20.9 Maintain the level of health you need to carry out your professional role.

20.10 Use all forms of spoken, written and digital communication (including social media and networking sites) responsibly, respecting the right to privacy of others at all times.

Being a member of the nursing profession is something to be proud of. Registering with the NMC at the end of your training is just the beginning of a lifelong journey. We never stop learning. Learning about ourselves, learning from our patients, nursing practice changes over time; we learn new skills and participate in innovations and research. We have the opportunity to help shape the care we deliver to the people in our care, some of whom may be loved ones, friends and relatives.

SOCIAL MEDIA X
@BellePUNC

A professional requires having the necessary training, experience, and understanding in your line of work as well as the ability to conduct yourself with consideration, courtesy, and respect.

We care for people at their most vulnerable, a very privileged position to be in. Patients trust us to do our job correctly and take the very best care of them as if they were our own family. Upholding the principles of the NMC will ensure we do this to the best of our ability, as an individual nurse, as a team, as a profession. Balancing our personal lives to uphold these principles will, at times, be difficult and challenging. At these times, think about the notes you have made about what your profession means to you. It may help guide your reactions and responses to these difficult and challenging situations. Reflection is a powerful tool you learn during your nurse training, a lifelong skill you need to embed into your daily life. Reflection is a key component of the revalidation process that all nurses undertake every 3 years. Use the situations you are faced with for reflection. Discuss them with trusted colleagues, your mentors, your leaders. Keep a written account; they are useful to look back on when faced with similar situations.

> Think about how you behave inside and outside of the workplace. If you were to see a colleague behaving in the same way, what would you think? Does it portray professionalism? Would you feel confident that they know how to care for you when you are at your most vulnerable?
>
> _____
> _____
> _____
> _____
> _____
> _____

CONCLUSION

Be proud to be part of the nursing profession. Uphold the values and principles of the NMC code in everything that you do, and reflect daily. Achieving a balance between your personal and professional lives does get easier; it takes practice, and you will make some mistakes along the way. It is how you respond at the time and reflect and learn from them that matters.

Space for reader's own reflection:
_____
_____
_____
_____
_____
_____
_____
_____
_____
_____
_____
_____
_____
_____
_____
_____
_____
_____
_____

REFERENCES

Blau, A., Sela, Y., Grinberg, K., 2023. Public Perceptions and Attitudes on the Image of Nursing in the Wake of COVID-19. Int. J. Environ. Res. Public Health 20 (6), 4717.

Crown Prosecution Service. n.d. Drug offences [Online]. https://www.cps.gov.uk/crime-info/drug-offences [Accessed November 28, 2023]

ten Hoeve, Y., Jansen, G., Roodbol, P., 2014. The nursing profession: public image, self-concept and professional identity. A discussion paper. J. Adv. Nurs [Online] 70 (2), 295–309.

Ghadirian, F., Salsali, M., Cheraghi, M.A. 2014. Nursing professionalism: An evolutionary concept analysis. Iran J. Nurs. Midwifery Res. 19 (1), 1−10.

Griffith, R., 2013. Ethical dilemmas in nursing. Br. J. Nurs 22 (18), 1087. https://www-magonlinelibrary-com.ezproxy.uwe.ac.uk/doi/full/10.12968/bjon.2013.22.18.1087 [Accessed February 11, 2024]

Nursing and Midwifery Council. 2023. The Code Professional standards of practice and behaviour for nurses, midwives and nursing associates [Online]. https://www.nmc.org.uk/globalassets/sitedocuments/nmc-publications/nmc-code.pdf [Accessed November 28, 2023]

Nursing and Midwifery Council. 2023. Our role [Online]. Nursing and Midwifery Council https://www.nmc.org.uk/about-us/our-role/ [Accessed March 23, 2024]

Nursing and Midwifery Council. 2024. Understanding fitness to practise: Fitness to practise allegations - Misconduct [Online]. https://www.nmc.org.uk/ftp-library/understanding-fitness-to-practise/fitness-to-practise-allegations/misconduct/ [Accessed March 23, 2024]

Oxford Languages. 2024. Ethical dilemma meaning [Online]. https://www.google.com/search?sca_esv=100a8d72724cfbcd&rlz=1CAZVTZ_enGB935GB935&q=ethical+dilemma&si=AKbGX_qbffDhNJNmNuoQO9DPv_17dXNUWsRYP-sMZiKRrGd8WrmVuZowvUoJyFHOd2QAz4dvQRysSkZQVrYh5QLmGgCpdTormGCT0B7CpwA-XsIjE1rI-QU%3D&expnd=1&sa=X&ved=2ahUKEwi87cv-14qFAxUJQkEAHUjwBX4Q2v4IegQIHhAS&biw=1396&bih=632&dpr=1.38 [Accessed March 23, 2024.

Raines, M.L. 2000. Ethical decision making in nurses: Relationships among moral reasoning, coping style, and ethics stress. Jona's Healthc. Law Ethics Regul 2, 29–41.

Remshardt, M. 2012. Do you know your professional boundaries? Nurs. Made Incredibly Easy! 10 (1), 5−6.

Royal College of Nursing. 2024. Definition and Principles of Nursing [Online]. Royal College of Nursing. https://www.rcn.org.uk/Professional-Development/Definition-and-Principles-of-Nursing[Accessed March 23, 2024.

Royal College of Nursing. 2022. UK nursing confirmed as most trusted profession as strike risk grows [Online]. https://www.rcn.org.uk/news-and-events/news/uk-nursing-confirmed-as-most-trusted-profession-as-strike-risk-grows-231122 [Accessed March 23, 2024]

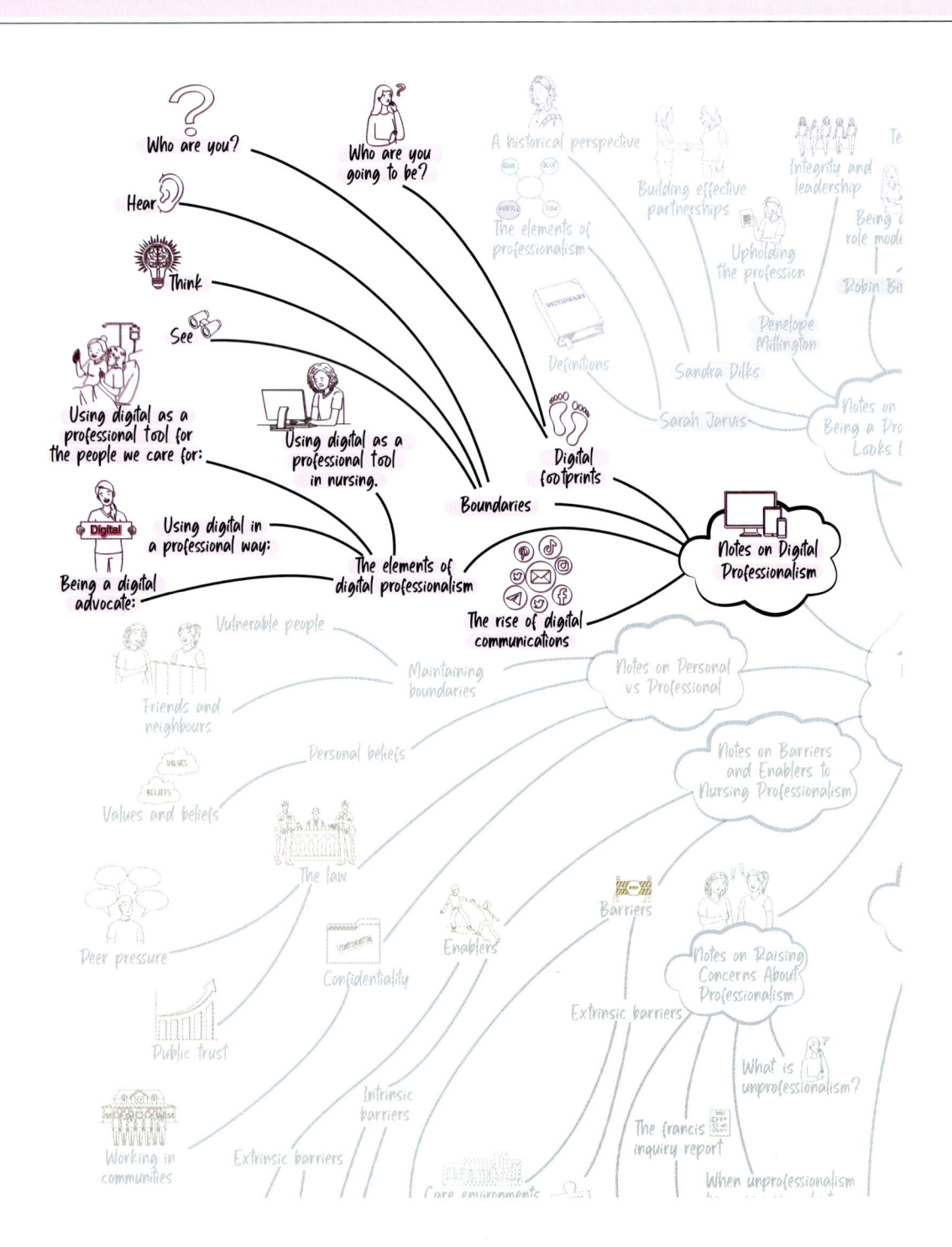

Notes on Digital Professionalism

- Who are you?
- Who are you going to be?
- Hear
- Think
- See
- Using digital as a professional tool for the people we care for:
- Using digital as a professional tool in nursing.
- Using digital in a professional way:
- Being a digital advocate:
- The elements of digital professionalism
- Boundaries
- Digital footprints
- The rise of digital communications

7

NOTES ON DIGITAL PROFESSIONALISM

Teresa Chinn (she/her)

INTRODUCTION

As the use of digital and social media has risen, so has the need for registered nurses, nursing associates and nursing students to understand digital professionalism. Although there is no standard definition for digital professionalism, the term has emerged in response to the need for health professionals (including registered nurses, nursing associates and midwives) to understand, develop and know appropriate professional behaviour when using digital media (Mather and Cummings 2019). This chapter explores the concept of digital professionalism, what it means for nursing students and how nursing students can be digitally professional.

THE RISE OF DIGITAL COMMUNICATIONS

In 1971, the first ever email was sent (Swatman 2015); however, the introduction of email into the NHS was not until 2002 (Heather 2016), and since then, digital communications in health and care have been snowballing, albeit at a sedate pace! Professional digital communication is a vital skill for all registered nurses, and today, digital communication, whether it is email, text messaging, apps, voice recordings (podcasts and voice notes), video recordings (YouTube and other videos), websites or social media, is here to stay and on the rise. In 2016, an average of 150 million emails and 20.8 million WhatsApp messages were sent… every minute!!!! (Visual Capitalist 2016). By 2021, internet use and digital communication increased significantly, with 197.6 million emails sent and 69 million messages sent via WhatsApp and Messenger (see image below)...*every minute*!!!! (European Commission 2021)

Digital has become a default way to communicate and an overwhelmingly important aspect of nursing. In 2009, Eric Qualman (a social media expert) stated, 'We no longer have a choice on whether we do social media, the question is how well we do it', and while the same can be said for wider digital communications, this is something that we are just realising within nursing. Digital is the way that a large proportion of the people we care for (and their families) communicate; therefore nursing students need to understand this method of communication and how to communicate in a digitally professional way.

WHY DIGITAL?

To understand digital professionalism and see the value of using digital spaces in nursing, we first need to understand why we should even contemplate using digital communication.

- What's in it for the people we care for?
- What's in it for us?
- What's in it for our teams and organisations?

In 2018, the Royal College of Nursing (RCN) published the findings of a consultation around the digital future of nursing that goes some way to answering these questions; they concluded that:

1. Better outcomes were needed for patients: that data, information, knowledge and technology had the potential to improve services for people receiving care so that they had better experiences and achieved better health and well-being outcomes.
2. Better experiences were needed for staff: the working lives of nurses and midwives could be improved through data, information, knowledge and technology, enabling people to experience increased levels of satisfaction and empowerment in their roles.
3. More efficient ways of working were needed: nursing and midwifery care could be delivered more efficiently, and in the best cases, a digitally enabled health service would free nurses and

7 | NOTES ON DIGITAL PROFESSIONALISM

midwives to devote more time to the people and populations who need their services.

Digital communications have the potential to provide better outcomes for the people we care for and improve registered nurses' working lives and ultimately deliver a better service.

In addition to this, the Queen's Nursing Institute (QNI)'s report (2023), 'Nursing in the Digital Age 2023', highlights the importance of digital technologies in nursing (specifically community nursing) and states that nurses have an 'appetite for high functioning technology and can see the potential of new applications, for example in managing wound care or long-term conditions. Indeed, some members of the community nursing workforce have taken an active part in the design of local solutions'. The QNI recommends that nurses should be involved at an early stage in the design and development of software and systems.

Digital communication is an integral part of nursing and a part that nurses are embracing, and because of this, registered nurses, nursing associates and nursing students need to be digitally aware and competent as nurses and aware of the importance of digital technology and communication in nursing.

SOCIAL MEDIA X
@Golding_PUNC22

'With regards to healthcare, professionalism translates into a digital space because it enables communication between staff members if face to face interaction isn't possible. It is also an effective way of exchanging ideas and important information'.

SOCIAL MEDIA X
@PUNC22NicMcMaho

'Professionalism translates into a digital space by remembering that clocking off does not mean clocking out professionally, we remain professional in and out of uniform, therefore always need to be mindful before posting on social media #PUNC22'

THE ELEMENTS OF DIGITAL PROFESSIONALISM

Chinn (n.d.) identifies four elements of digital professionalism:

- being a digital advocate;
- using digital in a professional way;
- using digital as a professional tool for the people we care for;
- using digital as a professional tool in nursing.

Each of these elements overlaps and intertwines, but they collectively make up what a good digitally professional registered nurse role model looks like. A good way to truly understand the different aspects of digital professionalism in nursing is via these four elements:

Being a digital advocate: It's important that registered nurses, nursing associates and nursing students promote digital technology and its use in health, act as leaders for the digital agenda, use digital technology with competence, champion digital technology and communication with the people they care for, and be a digital role model to others.

> **THE NMC SAYS**
>
> **20.8** Act as a role model of professional behaviour for students and newly qualified nurses, midwives and nursing associates to aspire to.

The following case study shows how learning about digital professionalism early on can help registered nurses become digital advocates.

> **CASE STUDY**
>
> Julie is a newly qualified registered nurse. At the very start of Julie's nursing journey, she was introduced to digital professionalism by her university. The university's digital professionalism module explored

CASE STUDY—cont'd

all aspects of digital communication and the use of technology in nursing. Throughout her time as a nursing student, Julie found that she was able to weave digital professionalism into being a nursing student, and once she had qualified, this became part of the way she worked. Some of the things with which Julie demonstrates digital professionalism in her day-to-day work include:

- Julie connects in social media spaces in a professional way and acts as role model to others.
- Julie frequently advocates apps and technology to the people she cares for.
- Julie uses all forms of digital communication in a responsible and professional way.
- Julie takes what she learns in digital spaces and share it with others as needed, including the people she cares for.
- Julie spends time with nursing students, explaining digital professionalism.

While on X (formerly Twitter) one day, Julie learns about All Our Health, a framework of evidence from the Office for Health Improvement and Disparities (2015) to guide healthcare professionals in preventing illness, protecting health and promoting well-being. Julie takes some time to have a look at the resource and explore; she is particularly interested in the cardiovascular disease prevention section, as this is her area of work. While exploring, Julie notices some examples of good practice from her local area, in particular, a walking group for people who have experienced cardiovascular problems. Julie starts to use this knowledge in her practice and tell the people she cares for about the group. Julie also starts to advocate the All Our Health digital resource to colleagues and nursing students.

Julie not only promotes and advocates digital in nursing but also takes what she learns and finds and uses it to improve the lives of the people she cares for.

> **TIPS**
> A great place to start to become a digital advocate in nursing is to join X. There are lots of nurses who are passionate about digital and digital professionalism using X to share information, resources and ideas and to hold discussions. Some interesting hashtags to take a look at include:
>
> #WeNurses
> #AllOurHealth
> #NewNotesOnNursing
> #TeamCNO

Using digital in a professional way: Registered nurses and nursing students should be digitally literate; be approachable, respectful and honest in digital communications; and practice in line with the NMC code of conduct (NMC 2018) and NMC social media guidance (NMC 2019).

> **THE NMC SAYS**
> 20.10 Use all forms of spoken, written and digital communication (including social media and networking sites) responsibly, respecting the right to privacy of others at all times.

The following case study below explores how digital communications can come across as unprofessional:

> **CASE STUDY**
> Sandy is a newly qualified registered nurse who has been qualified for less than a year and works as a practice nurse in a GP surgery. Sandy's manager asks them to come in for a meeting regarding a Facebook comment that Sandy has posted on the surgery's Facebook page. The comment is in response to a post about the

7 | NOTES ON DIGITAL PROFESSIONALISM

> **CASE STUDY—cont'd**
>
> surgery's asthma clinic, and Sandy uses a swear word in the comment. Sandy's manager asks them to reflect on the post, particularly in relation to the NMC code of conduct. When Sandy rereads the Facebook comment, they decide to delete it, and they reflect that their manager has raised an important issue, as, on this occasion, the comment was not digitally professional, and Sandy's communication came across as disrespectful. The manager and Sandy have a reflective discussion around respectful communication and how sometimes people can forget that social media spaces are public facing.

In this case study, Sandy reflects that their comment is not professional on this occasion, but it's important to realise that digital professionalism, as with professionalism, is not an exact science. What one person sees as being unprofessional, others may see as being professional, so it's important to look and reflect on professionalism, including digital professionalism, from all perspectives. It's important to also remember that digital professionalism isn't just about the written word, as in the case study here, but it extends to photos, videos and voice recordings, so care needs to be taken regardless of the media.

> What are your thoughts on the case study shown here? Do you see swear words on a social media post as being digitally unprofessional, or are there times when this is respectful and okay?
>
> _____
> _____
> _____
> _____

Using digital tools, media and communication in a professional way can mean different things to different people, but there are times when it is obvious that a registered nurse, nursing associate or nursing student is being unprofessional. The NMC social media guidance (NMC 2019) states that 'Nurses, midwives and nursing associates may put their registration at risk, and students may jeopardise their ability to join our register, if they act in any way that is unprofessional or unlawful on social media including (but not limited to):

- sharing confidential information inappropriately
- posting pictures of patients and people receiving care without their consent
- posting inappropriate comments about patients
- bullying, intimidating or exploiting people
- building or pursuing relationships with patients or service users
- stealing personal information or using someone else's identity
- encouraging violence or self-harm
- inciting hatred or discrimination'.

TIPS

Tips for using digital communications in a professional way:

- Spend some time observing how other registered nurses, nursing associates and nursing students behave in digital environments, including emails, social media and forums.
- Remember that digital communications are permanent: even if you have the ability to delete once sent, someone may have taken a screenshot or picture of your communication, so always reread and sense check before hitting send.
- If in doubt, think about your digital communication/behaviour using a 'real-world' analogy; If you wouldn't do it in the 'real world', then perhaps you should not do it in a digital space.
- If you are annoyed, angry, drunk or very tired, remember that digital communication devices have an off button, and step away!
- If in doubt, phone a friend—though, to be honest, if you have enough doubts to phone a friend, then you probably already know!

> **TIPS—cont'd**
> - Remember it's okay to disagree with people; just disagree politely.
> - Remember that the vast majority of registered nurses, nursing associates and nursing students are digitally professional—so have some confidence, too!

Using digital as a professional tool for the people we care for: Registered nurses and nursing students should explore how they can use digital communication and technology to connect with and care for people, they should use digital as part of their core work and not as an add-on or afterthought, they should be aware of what digital technology is available and how it can support people, and they should be mindful of maintaining professional boundaries.

> **THE NMC SAYS**
>
> **20.6** Stay objective and have clear professional boundaries at all times with people in your care (including those who have been in your care in the past), their families and carers.

> 'I have been very fortunate throughout my career to have opportunities to progress, whatever speciality of nursing or employer, NHS or voluntary, charity, social enterprise, and now working at the Queens Nursing Institute. Progress has included developing knowledge and skills working with the digital agenda and understanding the real difference it can make but recognizing, too, we must not exclude those people who for various reasons do not have access, the skills, the finances and seek to support those as best we can; knowing how to and if we don't, ensuring we know who can while remembering and advocating a personalised approach to those who do not want to engage in the digital world, asking "what matters to you".

Continued

Digital professionalism is no different to me than professionalism in other areas of nursing, and in recent years, (I) have had the privilege to lead several digital projects, including an app, films, e-cookbook and digital billboard, and (I) volunteer for two nursing charities, supporting their social media. Digital professionalism is underpinned by the Code (NMC 2018), prioritising people, practising effectively, preserving safety and promoting professionalism and trust. Leading a project coproducing resources with young carers demonstrated this to me. Young carers were offered the opportunity to take part in a project where they were invited to share their lived experience and make a film to share their experiences to raise awareness of young carers. The young carers were always treated with respect and given choices, and the project went at their pace. They were excited to be filmed and know their films would be on YouTube and organisations' websites and have a national launch and webinar. When being promoted, the films would be on social media, too. Consent was vital awareness they knew what platforms their films would be hosted on and who the target and audience was. Practising effectively was demonstrated through the leadership of the project and the finished result of a series of short films. As the project manager with a compassionate and participative leadership style, listening to and collaborating with the young carers and the multiagency project team was essential, and this was online, ensuring there was time at the end of meetings to debrief if needed and being aware that if people had their cameras off, were they okay? Time was spent with a parent concerned about her child being on social media but, at the end of the project, was promoting the films herself on Facebook! Preserving safety was essential

Celebration events were face to face; all meetings, engagement sessions and editing were online, either Zoom or MS Teams. I ensured the young carers always had a young carers worker on the call too, someone they knew, someone who could step in or reach out to them when they were sharing their stories if they became upset (and this did happen one occasion). Promoting professionalism and trust was demonstrated through ensuring at all times I was professional and aware of professional boundaries, using appropriate language when

7 | NOTES ON DIGITAL PROFESSIONALISM

leading engagement sessions, Tweeting about the progress of the project, chairing webinars to launch the film nationally or writing blogs.

I am proud to be a nurse, and being professional is important to me and inherent in my practice, wherever I've worked. Leading digital projects is exciting, and although nervous at first, on reflection, (I) recognise the myriad of transferable skills I, as a nurse, brought, including teamwork, communication, people skills, organisational skills, decision making, problem solving. I have seen firsthand the positive difference digital projects can make to people and stakeholders, and this extends to me, too!'

Fiona Rogers, RN, SCPHN, SN, QN

TIPS

Don't see digital as an add-on to being a registered nurse but simply as being part of nursing.

Using digital as a professional tool for nurses: Registered nurses, nursing associates and nursing students should explore and be aware of the use of digital technology and communication to aid with reflection, discussion and idea sharing, to connect with evidence and research, to aid with professional development, and to network with others.

THE NMC SAYS

Practise effectively: You assess need and deliver or advise on treatment, or give help (including preventative or rehabilitative care) without too much delay and to the best of your abilities, on the basis of the best evidence available and best practice. You communicate effectively, keeping clear and accurate records and sharing skills, knowledge and experience where appropriate. You reflect and act on any feedback you receive to improve your practice.

Digital communication and technology are not just about the people we care for, and part of being a digitally professional nurse is being able to use digital to support ourselves. There is a lot of potential for digital to support the way we work, learn, get support and reflect in nursing. The following case study explores just one way in which this can be done.

> **CASE STUDY**
>
> Steffan is a registered nurse who has been qualified for just under 3 years and is due to revalidate for the very first time. Since qualifying, Steffan has been writing a reflective blog of his nursing journey. Steffan's blogs are public, and he keeps his reflections generic and nonspecific so that he does not breach confidentiality in any way. Steffan encourages and joins in the discussion that other people post as comments on his blog and finds this useful as part of reflective practice. When the time comes to revalidate, Steffan is able to use his reflective blog posts as reflections for his revalidation.

In this case study, Steffan uses his blog to support his reflective practice and his revalidation, but in the context of being digitally professional, there is so much more that registered nurses, nursing associates and nursing students can do in regard to using digital as a professional tool. The following tip box explores a few more ideas.

> **TIPS**
>
> Supporting revalidation and reflective practice in digital spaces:
>
> - Reflection: Start a blog, vlog or podcast to reflect on practice. Remember to keep reflections generic, and respect confidentiality.
> - Discussion: Join in a discussion on X; a good place to start is #WeNurses, which is usually on a Thursday evening.
> - Idea sharing: Be generous with your ideas in digital spaces, and ask others for their ideas and thoughts. Get involved in forums, Facebook groups and discussions on X.

> **TIPS—cont'd**
> - **Connecting with evidence and research:** Follow accounts such as Cochrane, WHO, National Institute for Health and Care Excellence (NICE), Office for Health Improvement and Disparities (OHID) and NHS England on social media. Engage with the research and evidence they share, and share interesting things you find, too.
> - **Professional development:** Think about professional development and learning differently. Learning doesn't always come from a classroom; it can be something you read in a blog that made you think, such as a really interesting YouTube video or even an email discussion with your practice supervisor.
> - **Networking with others:** Networking no longer has to be face to face; email, forums, webinars and social media are all great ways to expand your network. Start to think of your network as a group of experts who can support you through your nursing journey, and get your virtual networking game on!

THE NMC AND DIGITAL PROFESSIONALISM

It's important to remember that whatever the setting—in real-life or digital settings—the code is not negotiable or discretionary and applies to *all settings* as a standard for practice and behaviour. Being digitally professional as a nurse is about taking the code and applying it to our digital spaces.

> **THE NMC SAYS**
>
> **20.10** Use all forms of spoken, written and digital communication (including social media and networking sites) responsibly, respecting the right to privacy of others at all times.

The NMC (DATE) has also produced specific guidance on the use of social media entitled 'Guidance on using social media responsibly', and this is essential reading for all nursing students. The guidance 'is not intended to cover every social media situation, however it sets out principles to enable nurses to think through issues and act professionally, ensuring public protection at all times'.

Being a professional and being a digital professional isn't something that you can clock in and clock out of; being professional is a way of life as a nurse and equally so as a nurse in a digital space. The NMC has a series of videos that can be found on their website, entitled 'Caring with Confidence'. All of the videos are worth watching; however, the 'Let's talk about professionalism' video explores professionalism specifically and states that being a professional takes into account behaviours, knowledge, excellence, integrity, role modelling and more. Furthermore, the video explains how these things are not just for when you are working and need to be taken into account when not working, too. The 'Lets talk about social media' video in the series expands on this by stating that although your social media post may have nothing to do with your role as a registered nurse, nursing associate or midwife, anything you share can affect your professional reputation.

BOUNDARIES

Professional boundaries are a large part of staying digitally professional. Cooper and Inglehearn (2015) introduce the concept of 'context collapse', which can lead to challenges for professionals and challenges with maintaining digital professionalism. Cooper and Inglehearn explain that in day-to-day life, communication occurs in a context where we can see it and make sense of it, and they give an example: 'healthcare professionals acting in a caring role with patients can generally understand the context of that communication and interaction. They may behave differently if they see the same person later in a social context such as out shopping'. These interactions have boundaries, and there is an understanding of the professional behaviour expected. Digital communication, however, creates an environment where communication happens within multiple contexts and often with none of the subtle clues, body language and intonation of speech that face-to-face contact creates, and the context of the communication is lost, leaving the recipient of the communication to fill in the gaps. This can lead to miscommunications and misunderstandings and provides a challenge for registered nurses, nursing associates and nursing students. Cooper and Inglehearn express how context can help professionals to make interactions professional and safe and that the lack of context can put a strain on professional boundaries.

Professional boundaries are a huge part of being digitally professional, as they help to define what is expected and what is acceptable; they protect the people we care for and the public but are also vital in ensuring that registered nurses, nursing associates and nursing students do not get burnt out and that they enjoy lengthy careers (Day-Calder 2016). In order to maintain boundaries, especially in the light of context collapse, Cooper and Inglehearn (2015) suggest that registered nurses 'see, think and act' in regard to their digital selves, and they advise that registered nurses ask themselves a series of reflective questions around their digital personas; these are explored in Fig. 7.1.

Think about how you can apply 'see, think and act' to your practice:
_____
_____
_____
_____
_____

DIGITAL FOOTPRINTS

Google (2024) describes a digital footprint as 'the information about a particular person that exists on the internet as a result of their online activity'. Being aware and mindful of your digital footprint is a major part of digital professionalism. It's important to be aware of what you look

NURSING PROFESSIONALISM FOR NURSING STUDENTS

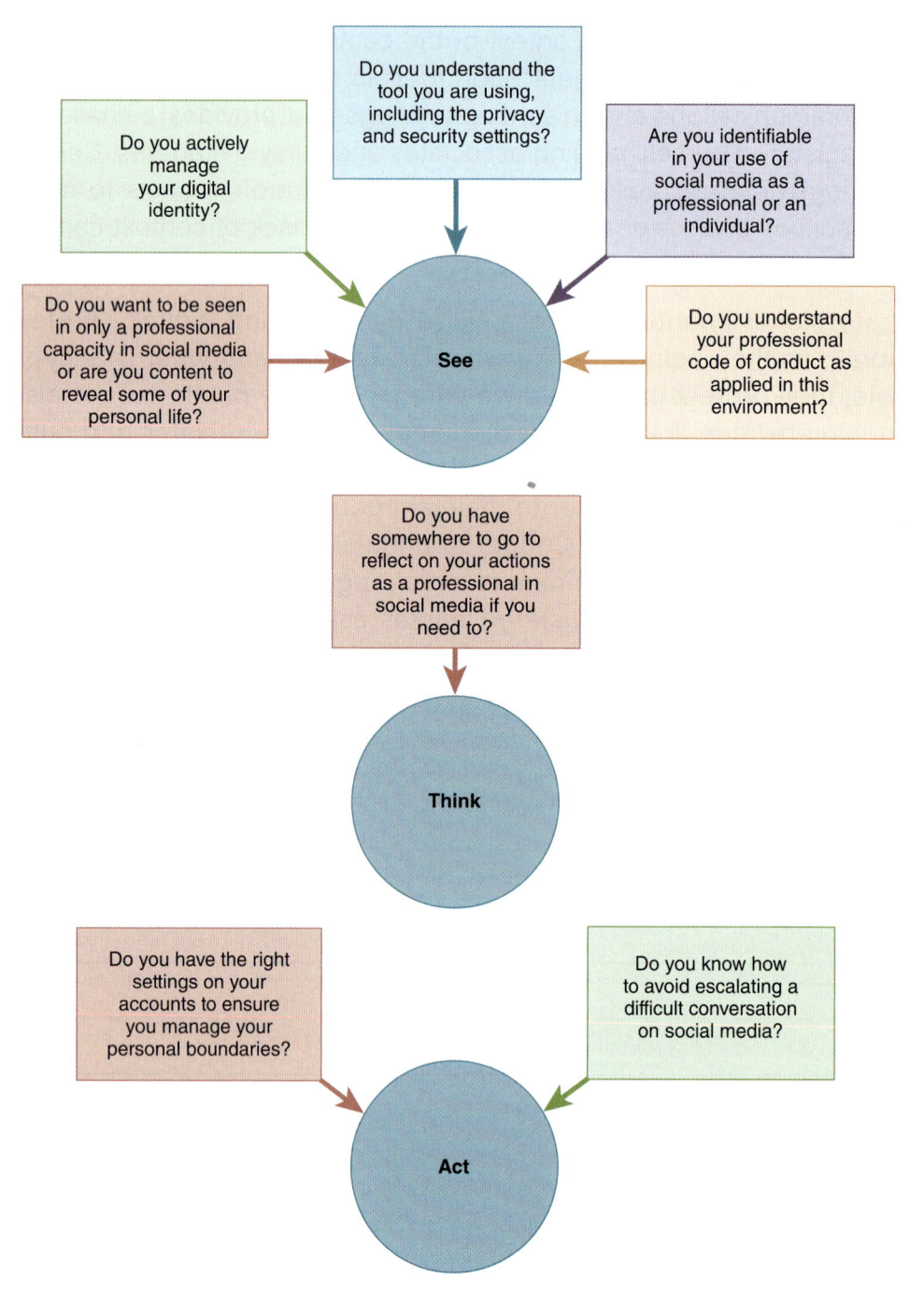

See
- Do you understand the tool you are using, including the privacy and security settings?
- Do you actively manage your digital identity?
- Are you identifiable in your use of social media as a professional or an individual?
- Do you want to be seen in only a professional capacity in social media or are you content to reveal some of your personal life?
- Do you understand your professional code of conduct as applied in this environment?

Think
- Do you have somewhere to go to reflect on your actions as a professional in social media if you need to?

Act
- Do you have the right settings on your accounts to ensure you manage your personal boundaries?
- Do you know how to avoid escalating a difficult conversation on social media?

Figure 7.1 I see, think, and act.

7 | NOTES ON DIGITAL PROFESSIONALISM

like in a digital space and how others may perceive you, both in order to ensure you are not doing anything wrong that may lead to breaking the NMC code and in order to ensure that you are doing things right and this is visible to people.

> ### SOCIAL MEDIA X
> **@indiaxpunc22**
>
> 'Remembering you always leave a digital footprint so to always be mindful. Remember to respect patient privacy & what you say can be taken in different ways, so also remember that when posting .. be your best professionalism self!!'

It's important to understand that digital footprints are not a bad thing; in fact, they can be a very good thing! One of the most amazing things about digital footprints is that you are in control of them and you can shape them into what you want them to be. The sketch note in Fig. 7.2 explores digital footprints a little more, particularly the idea that you are in control of your digital footprint and it can be a positive thing to take forward in your nursing career:

> Take 5 minutes to Google yourself—what do you see? If you don't see anything, try adding your location as well as your name. Do you like what you see?
> _____
> _____
> _____
> _____
> _____

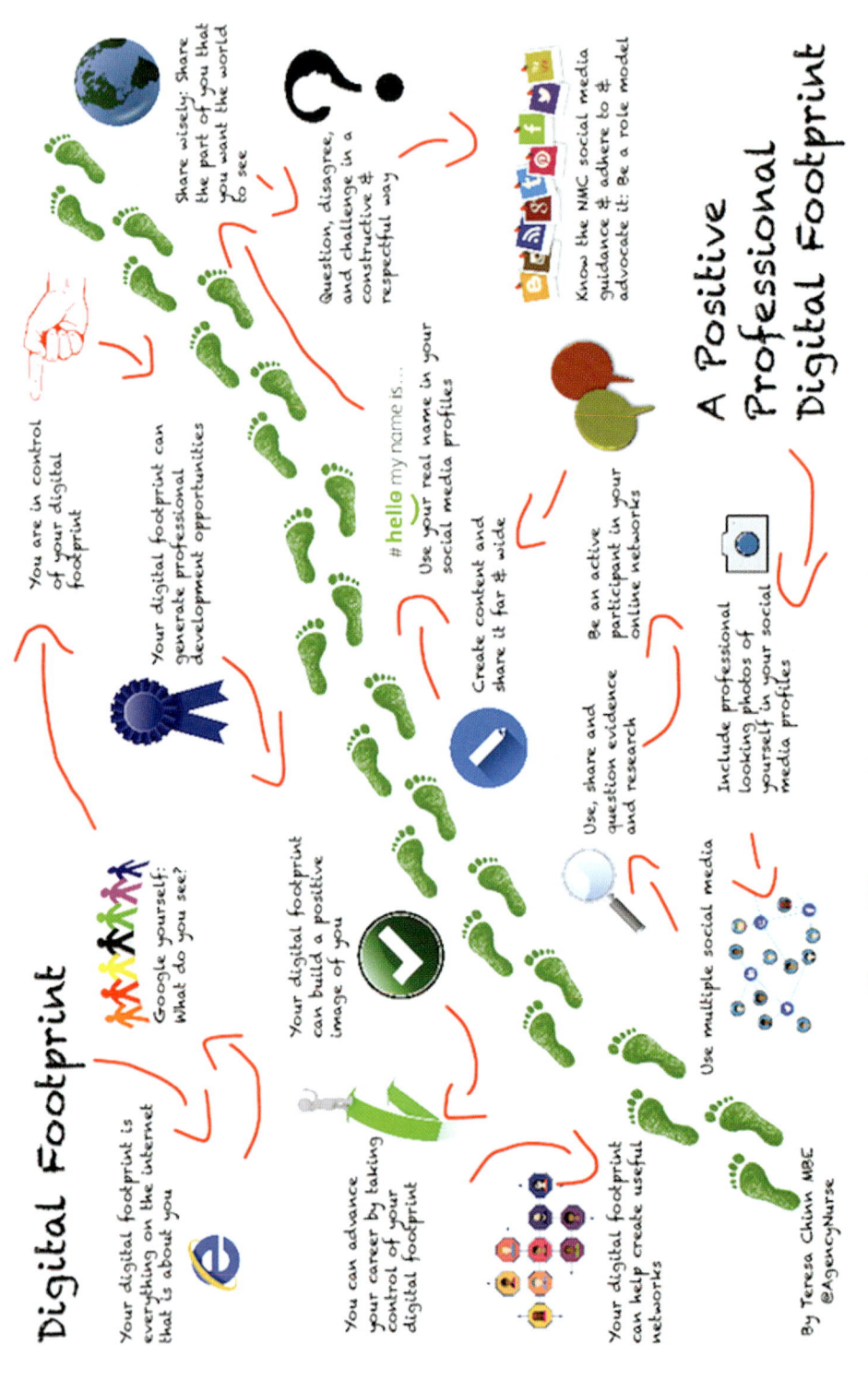

Figure 7.2 A positive professional digital footprint.

The University of Edinburgh (2016) identifies two key questions when it comes to digital footprints: 'who are you (now)?' and 'who are you going to be (in the future)?'

Who are you (now)?

- What does your digital footprint look like right now?
- Is your current digital footprint an accurate representation of you?
- If someone Googled you, what would they find?
- Would this be beneficial or a potential disadvantage for working as a nurse?
- Does your online profile(s) describe you in a personal or professional context?
- Is your online presence accurate and up to date?

Who are you going to be (in the future)?

- What information do you want someone to find when they search for you in digital spaces?
- Do you want to keep your professional and personal identities separate, or do you want to blend them together?
- If you have multiple online identities on different platforms, is it obvious that they belong to you?

It's a good thing to ask yourself these questions, not just now at the start of your career but also from time to time as you go through your career.

THE POTENTIAL VERSUS THE RISKS

Digital professionalism is not just about what you don't do (i.e., not posting inappropriately, not using digital media to bully or harass), but it is also about taking positive steps and exploring the potential of digital spaces and media and how it can help you to be a professional. The NMC (DATE) states that 'if used responsibly and appropriately, social networking sites can offer several benefits for nurses, midwives, nursing associates, and students'. Fig. 7.3 outlines the benefits described by the NMC.

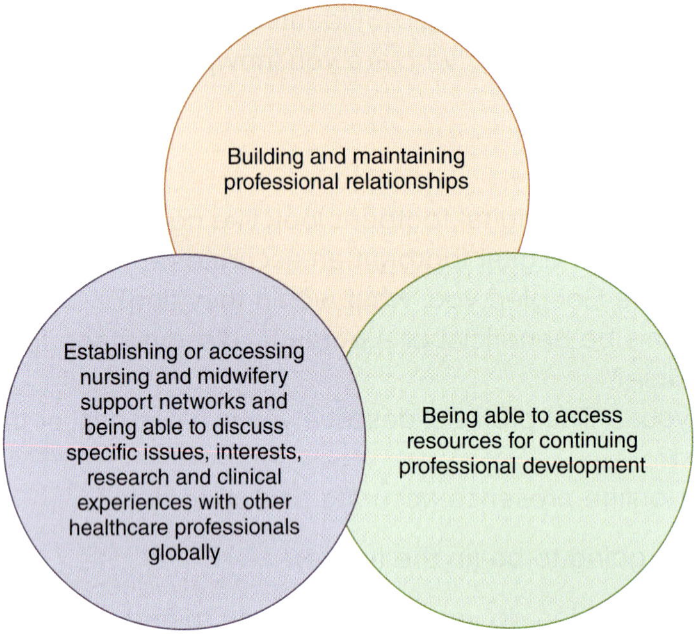

Figure 7.3 The benefits of social networking sites.

- Building and maintaining professional relationships
- Establishing or accessing nursing and midwifery support networks and being able to discuss specific issues, interests, research and clinical experiences with other healthcare professionals globally
- Being able to access resources for continuing professional development

Social and digital media can be incredibly positive and useful for nursing students, and the NMC recognises that taking steps to realise the potential is a positive thing for nursing. Ferguson (2013) builds on this and states: 'Embracing new technology requires a careful appraisal of "fit for purpose". However, sadly, the information revolution is being obstructed by those who have not carefully engaged in discussion and debate, but rather applied a lens of scepticism, risk aversion, and obstruction.' Fergusson identifies several barriers to adoption of social media in particular (but some can be applied to digital as a whole); these are outlined in Fig. 7.4.

Digital professionalism takes thought and courage, as, at its heart, it's about taking positive steps to realise the potential that digital has in nursing. In Fig. 7.5, Chinn (2020) identifies five ways in which nurses can start to unlock the potential of social media in nursing (as with Fergusson, this can also be applied to digital as a whole).

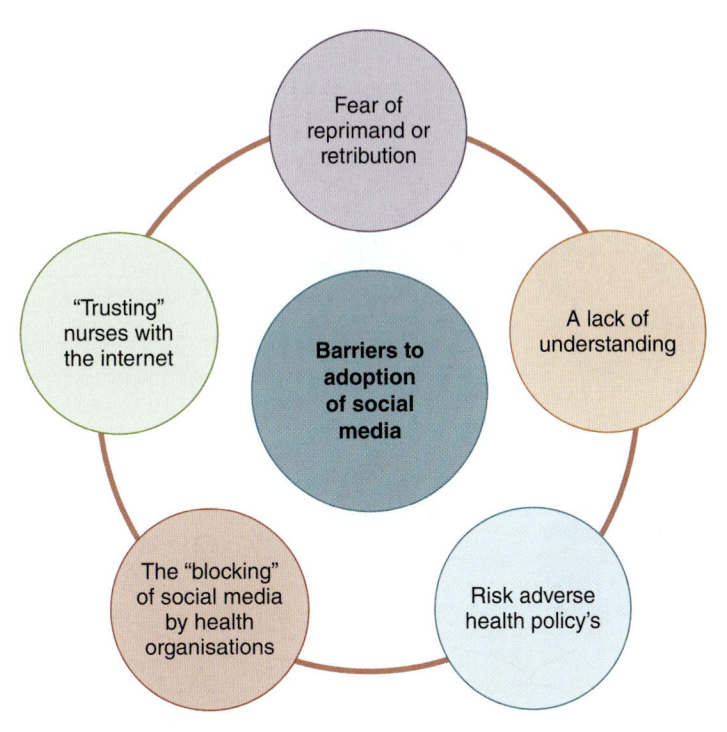

Figure 7.4 Barriers to the adoption of social media.

- Fear of reprimand or retribution
- "Trusting" nurses with the internet
- A lack of understanding
- The "blocking" of social media by health organisations
- Risk adverse health policy's
- Barriers to adoption of social media

McGrath et al. (2019) identifies that there are 'significant benefits of using social media for nursing students, such as developing professional networks, engaging in the nursing community, accessing and providing support, and enhancing their knowledge. However, nursing students must be made aware of the potential risks in relation to how they share information and communicate online'. It is important that when communicating online as a nursing student, even if you don't identify yourself, all interactions are professional. The risk of not communicating in a professional way is that nursing students may find that they are subject to misconduct investigations, which could result in exclusion from studies and being unable to join the professional register (McGrath et al. 2019). Nevertheless, the answer here is not as simple as not engaging in digital communication, as so much can be gained for both nursing students and the people they care for; the answer is to be smart. The following tips box outlines some strategies to help mitigate the risks of digital and online communication.

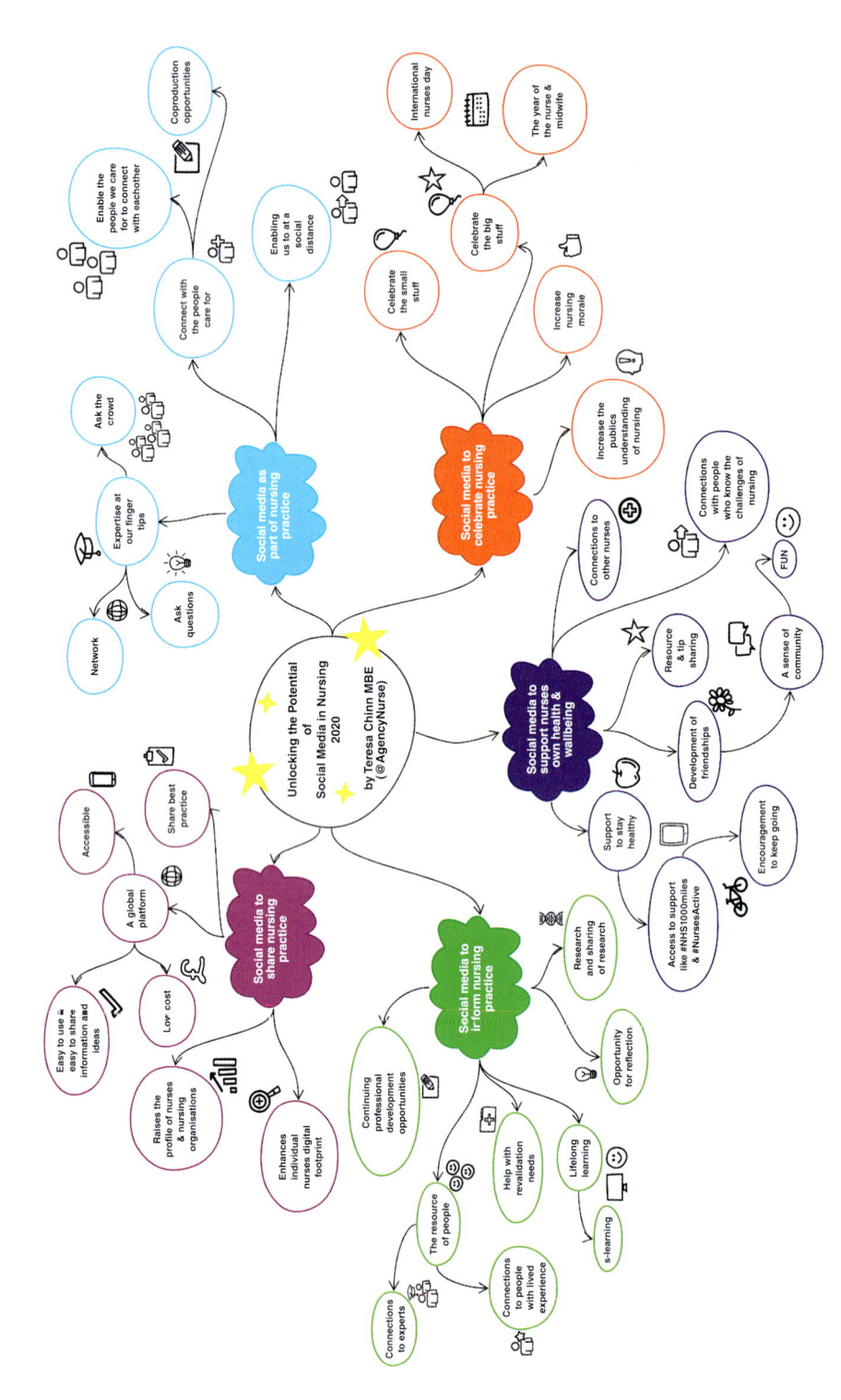

184 NURSING PROFESSIONALISM FOR NURSING STUDENTS

Figure 7.5 Unlocking the potential of social media in nursing.

TIPS

Online and digital communication can be tricky. Here are some things that may help:

- Just because social media and digital communication is instant doesn't mean you don't have. You can take time to think, phone a friend and then respond.
- If you feel angry, annoyed or upset, then don't hit send/post—go out for a walk, chat to a friend, colleague or mentor, or simply just turn your device off.
- Think of digital communication as communicating in a very public space—with a loudspeaker—if you wouldn't shout it from the highest rooftops, then don't hit send/post.
- Step away from all digital communications during and after consuming alcohol.
- Think carefully about posting pictures and videos—is there anything in the background that breaches confidentiality or could look unprofessional?
- Remember that you are a nursing student both offline and online and have to adhere to the NMC code of conduct.

Think about how you will reduce the risk of being unprofessional in your digital communications.

_____
_____
_____
_____
_____

EVIDENCE AND RESEARCH

Digital professionalism is about being open and receptive to all sorts of digital media and using it in a professional way to inform our practice and as part of the way we care for people. Being a digital professional means not just sharing things you find online with others online or compartmentalising your digital self and knowledge. It's about integrating it fully with your life as a nurse. Applying and sharing your knowledge with colleagues and the people you care for is a huge part of digital professionalism. As nurses, we must always practice in line with the best available evidence.

> **THE NMC SAYS**
>
> 6 Always practise in line with the best available evidence.

Part of being a digital professional is about:

- being aware of evidence and research around digital and how it impacts the people we care for,
- being aware of how you can use digital spaces to keep up to date with evidence and research,
- being aware how you can use digital spaces to share evidence and research, and
- being able to discuss the value of evidence and research constructively in digital spaces.

Digital evidence and research in healthcare is an exciting combination.

> **CASE STUDY**
>
> Cochrane UK (@CochraneUK on X) is using social media in an exemplary way to share evidence and research. Cochrane UK take important points of *Cochrane Reviews* (research) and boils them down to important points for practice and then put these into pictures, which they share on X, Instagram and Facebook. Cochrane UK also has a really informative blog

> **CASE STUDY—cont'd**
>
> called Evidently Cochrane. Cochrane UK also supports Students 4 Best Evidence, a network of students interested in evidence-based healthcare, which has a website with blogs and resources.

> **CASE STUDY**
>
> The@PUNC project is a great example of how social media can be used as part of research to improve healthcare and learning. Since 2014, Plymouth University has led the way in introducing nursing students to digital professionalism. Jones (2016) states 'The aim of the@PUNC project is that our students learn to be "digitally professional" and to take advantage of online discussions with other students, colleagues, and the public. Since October 2014, all first-year students have been introduced to the use of Twitter (X) and have been asked to set up their own Twitter (X) account'. The university encourages nursing students to engage in social media in a digitally professional way and holds discussions, quizzes and sharing on X as part of learning. King (2016) stated that as a result of the study, 'more than 70 per cent of students thought the inclusion of Twitter (X) was worthwhile, and the cohort also said they gained wider perspectives on nursing, better grasp of social media and broader understanding of topics such as health promotion'.

Another aspect of evidence and research and the digital agenda is related to academic work. From time to time, nursing students may find that they need to refer to something from a digital space in their academic work (though it's important to remember that a variety of references should always be used, and nursing students should always critically appraise the content, regardless of the source or style). The infographic in Fig. 7.6 outlines how you can do this with a few of the more popular types of social media you may wish to refer to—your librarian will be able to help you if you come across something on other forms of social media that aren't on this list.

NURSING PROFESSIONALISM FOR NURSING STUDENTS

Referencing in academic work (harvard style)

Twitter: Family Name, INITIAL (S) (or organisation). Year. *Full text of tweet*. [Twitter]. Day and month tweet posted. (Date accessed: Insert date). Available from: Insert URL

YouTube: Screen Name or Username. Year. *Title*. [Online] (Date Accessed: Insert date) Available from: Insert URL

Blogs: Family Name, INITIAL (S) (or organisation). Year. *Title of blog entry*. Date blog entry written. Title of blog. [Online] (Date Accessed: Insert date) Available from: Insert URL

Skype: Family Name, INITIAL (S) (of interviewee). Year. *Interview with (name of interviewee)*. Date. Location

Podcasts: Family Name, INITIAL (S) (of orginator). Year. *Title of episode*. Title of podcast. [Podcast] (Date accessed: Insert date) Available from: Insert URL/APP

Facebook: Family Name, INITIAL (S) (or organisation). Year. *Title of page*. [Facebook] Date post written (Date Accessed: Insert date) Available from: Insert URL

Figure 7.6 Referencing and social media.

CONCLUSION

Digital professionalism is an important part of nursing; it enables nurses to be able to see the benefits of digital communication and mitigate the risks in order to provide better care, and therefore it is something that nursing students need to understand and embrace. Being digitally professional is about understanding the NMC code of conduct (NMC 2019) and 'Guidance on using social media responsibly' (NMC DATE) and understanding professional boundaries and the elements of digital professionalism and applying this to practise. Ultimately, digital professionalism is not an additional extra to being a nursing student, and ultimately, as a nurse, it's a vital part of modern nursing.

7 | NOTES ON DIGITAL PROFESSIONALISM

Space for reader's own reflection:

REFERENCES

Chinn, T. 2020. It's been a while since I created the "Unlocking the Potential of Social Media in Nursing" mind map ... so here's a 2020 refresh .... with the inclusion of social media to support nurses own health & wellbeing:) [X] September 4. https://x.com/AgencyNurse/status/1301916667807772672?s=20 [Accessed January 23, 2024]

Chinn, T. n.d. The elements of digital professionalism. [Sketchnote] In: @WeNurses (2019) The elements of digital professionalism#TANTTT. [X] January 22. https://twitter.com/WeNurses/status/1087730685329264643 [Accessed January 23, 2024]

Cooper, A., Inglehearn, A., 2015. Managing professional boundaries and staying safe in digital spaces. J. Res. Nurs 20 (7), 625–633.

Day-Calder, M. 2016. Maintaining professional boundaries. Nurs. Stand. https://rcni.com/nursing-standard/careers/career-advice/maintaining-professional-boundaries-61286 [Accessed January 23, 2024]

European Commission. 2021. Title of webpage [Online]. https://ec.europa.eu/newsroom/rtd/items/713444/enhttps://ec.europa.eu/newsroom/rtd/items/713444/en [Accessed February 11, 2024]

Ferguson, C., 2013. It's time for the nursing profession to leverage social media. J. Adv. Nurs 69 (4), 745–747.

Google. 2024. Digital footprint definition. https://www.google.com/search?q=digital+footprint+definition&sca_esv=600376160&rlz=1CAZVTZ_enGB935GB935&ei=hz-uZdLaOa7ai-gPkMSFiA4&oq=digital+footprint+de&gs_lp=Egxnd3Mtd2l6LXNlcnAiFGRpZ2l0YWwgZm9vdHByaW50IGRlKgIIADIFEAAYgAQyBRAAGIAEMgUQABiABDIFEAAYgAQyBRAAGIAEMgUQABiABDIFEAAYgAQyBRAAGIAEMgUQABiABDIFEAAYgARIrhBQ-ANYzwhwAXgAkAEAmAFNoAGlAqoBATS4AQHIAQD4AQHCAgoQABhHGNYEGLADwgINEAAYgAQYigUYQxiA8lCChAAGlAEGIoFGEPCAg0QABiABBiKBRhDGLED4gMEGAAgYYgGAZAGCg&sclient=gws-wiz-serp [Accessed January 23, 2024]

Heather, B., 2016. NHSmail 2 rolled out to 200,000 NHS staff. Digital Health. https://www.digitalhealth.net/2016/06/nhsmail-2-rolled-out-to-200000-nhs-staff/#:~:text=NHSmail%202%20replaces%20the%20ageing,which%20was%20introduced%20in%202002 [Accessed January 23, 2024]

Jones, R., 2016. University of Plymouth Nursing Cohorts. University of Plymouth. https://www.plymouth.ac.uk/schools/school of-nursing-and-midwifery/punc [Accessed January 23, 2024]

King, A., 2016. Twitter should form part of the nursing curriculum, says new study. https://www.plymouth.ac.uk/news/study-suggests-twitter-should-be-in-nursing-curriculum [Accessed January 23, 2024]

Mather, C.A., Cummings, E., 2019. Developing and sustaining digital professionalism: a model for assessing readiness of healthcare environments and capability of nurses. BMJ Health Care Inform [Online] 26 [Accessed January 23, 2024]

McGrath, L., Swift, A., Clark, M., 2019. Understanding the benefits and risks of nursing students engaging with online social media. Nurs. Stand. 34 (10), 45–49.

Nursing and Midwifery Council. 2008. The code: Standards of conduct, performance and ethics for nurses and midwives. Nursing and Midwifery Council, London.

Nursing and Midwifery Council. 2019. Guidance on using social media responsibly. https://www.nmc.org.uk/globalassets/sitedocuments/nmc-publications/social-media-guidance.pdf [Accessed January 23, 2024]

Qualman, E., 2009. Socialnomics: How social media transforms the way we live and do business. John Wiley & Sons, New Jersey.

Royal College of Nursing. 2018. Every nurse is an e-nurse. https://www.rcn.org.uk/Professional-Development/Professional-services/Every-Nurse-an-eNurse [Accessed January 23, 2024]

Swatman, R., 2015. 1971: First ever email. Guinness World Records. https://www.guinnessworldrecords.com/news/60at60/2015/8/1971-first-ever-email-392973 [Accessed January 23, 2024]

The Queens Nursing Institute (2023) *Nursing in the digital age 2023*. Available from: https://qni.org.uk/wp-content/uploads/2023/02/Nursing-in-the-Digital-Age-2023.pdf [Accessed 23 January 2024]

University of Edinburgh. 2016. e-Professionalism. https://www.docs.hss.ed.ac.uk/iad/About_us/Digital_footprint/Student_eprofrofessionalism_guide_v1_2.pdf [Accessed January 23, 2024]

Visual Capitalist. 2016. What Happens in an Internet Minute (2016)? [Online]. https://www.visualcapitalist.com/what-happens-internet-minute-2016/#:~:text=Google%20literally%20processes%202.4%20million,of%20physical%20and%20digital%20goods

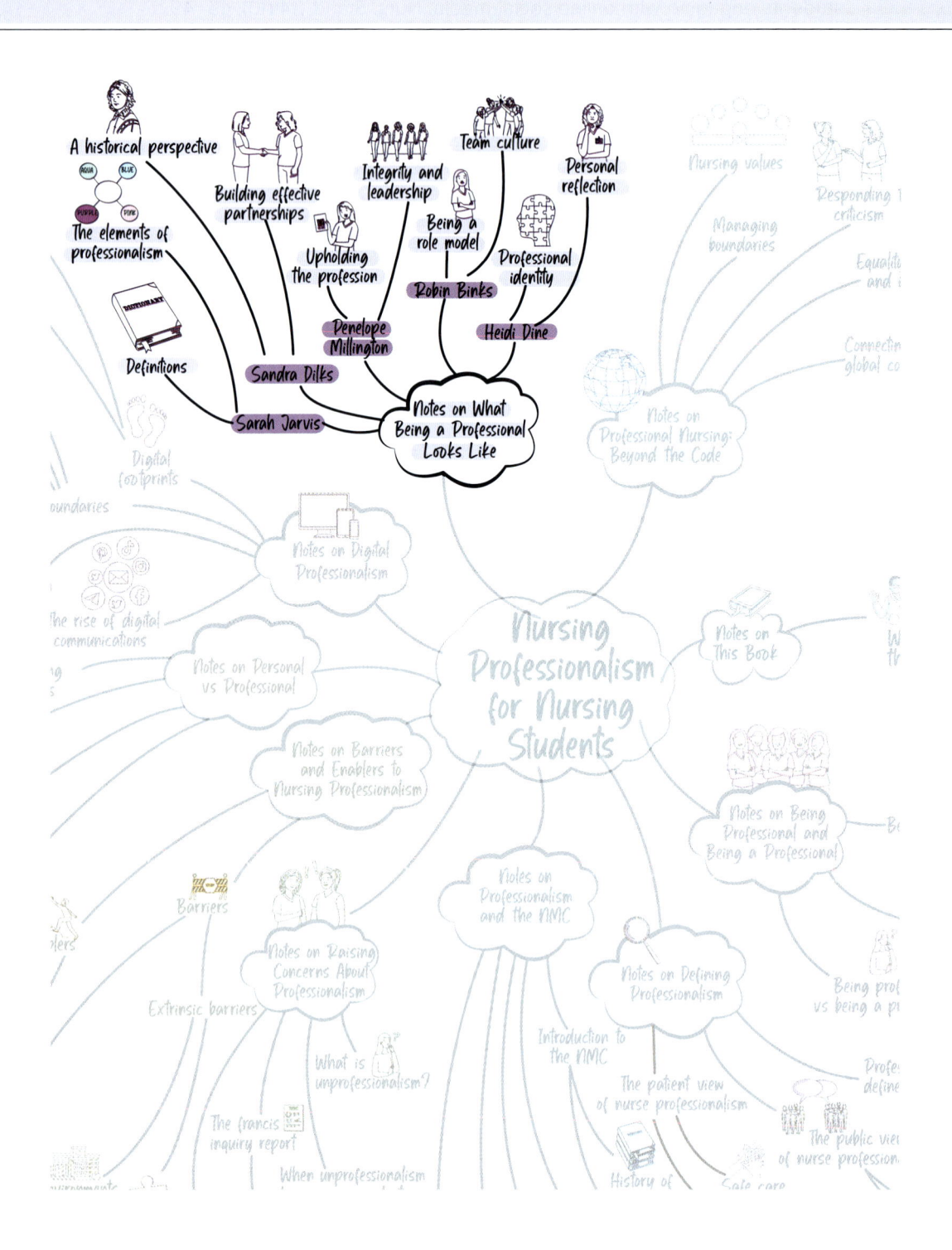

Notes on What Being a Professional Looks Like

- A historical perspective
- The elements of professionalism
- Definitions
- Sarah Jarvis
- Sandra Dilks
  - Building effective partnerships
  - Upholding the profession
- Penelope Millington
  - Integrity and leadership
  - Being a role model
- Robin Binks
  - Team culture
- Heidi Dine
  - Personal reflection
  - Professional identity

8

NOTES ON WHAT BEING A PROFESSIONAL LOOKS LIKE

Sarah Jarvis (she/her) ■ Sandra Dilks (she/her)
■ Penelope Millington ■ Robin Binks ■ Heidi Dine

INTRODUCTION

This chapter explores professionalism in nursing, considering what it is, what it means in practice and why it matters. The chapter has a range of authors, each bringing their own perspective on what being a professional looks like, but they are tied together with thoughts from Sarah Jarvis, who is an advanced clinical practitioner working in healthcare within the justice system.

As you embark on your student nursing journey and your nursing career, professionalism will be a pivotal part of this. Patients and families will place their trust in you, and fellow nursing colleagues and healthcare colleagues from other professional groups will look to you for inspiration and as a role model. In order to be the best you can be, your professional conduct will be key.

How you conduct yourself and the behaviour you display will be noticed by many. The impact your behaviour can and will have on others will be fundamental to the relationships you develop and how your career progresses. When things go wrong and nurses are investigated to assess their fitness to practice, it will often be due to their professional conduct coming into question or under dispute. When nurses let standards slip, this leads to them not adhering to the professional code of conduct. Understanding your own and others' professional conduct will help ensure you adhere to the Nursing and Midwifery Council (NMC) code.

Professionalism may appear to be obvious, which can lead to this topic not being explored in more detail; however, having a clear understanding of what it is will help you to be the most effective nurse you can be.

We will explore concepts around professionalism throughout this chapter to enable you to have greater confidence in being able to explain what professionalism is, the impact it has in practice and why it matters.

DEFINITIONS

What is professionalism?

The Oxford Dictionary definition of professionalism is:

> 'the high standard that you expect from a person who is well trained in a particular job'. (Oxford Learners Dictionary, n.d.)

As with any professional group, you would expect that nurses are trained to a high standard to carry out their role. As a nursing student, you will be undertaking a programme of study that will build your professional practice, where you will be given increasing responsibilities and opportunities to demonstrate your accountability. Once qualified, you will be supporting nursing students and junior colleagues in their roles by setting examples of how to practise.

> **Think of a person you admire and respect; this may be a nurse or another professional you have worked with on placement, or it could be a lecturer or teacher you admired. What is it about them that led you to admire this individual? What behaviours did they demonstrate?**
>
> _____
> _____
> _____
> _____

Sandra Dilks is an advanced clinical practitioner working as a senior lecturer within continuing professional development based at the University of Wolverhampton, leading the MSc advanced clinical practice programme. Qualifying in 2004, Sandra embarked on a career mainly focused in general practice, where she received the Queens Nurse Award in 2015. She joined the University of Wolverhampton in 2018, becoming a senior fellow of the Higher Education Academy, and she continues to have a passionate interest in the development of practice nurses while working as an external examiner for a general practice nurse preceptorship programme. In the next section, she not only defines professionalism but also explores the historical context when exploring what professionalism looks like to her.

SANDRA DILKS'S NOTES ON WHAT PROFESSIONALISM LOOKS LIKE

The first definition of 'profession' first began in the 19th century, and at this time, it was seen to encompass the need to focus on the importance of specialised skills, knowledge and competence guided by a code of ethics (Barton and Allan 2015). Although the concept of a professional occupation dates back farther to the 18th century, when it was believed there were only three great professions—godship, law and medicine—this sentiment continues. Fundamentally, health professionals continue this approach, as they have agreed-upon values and a code which may be set by the General Medical Council (GMC), Nursing and Midwifery Council (NMC) or the Health and Care Professions Council (HCPC). They are accountable to the larger society as representatives of their field of practice, and this is demonstrated through their behaviour and professionalism. However, when comparing the vision of professionalism in the 18th century to today's society, there is a greater distinction between professionalism related to behaviour and that of the notoriety of a status or financial gain from being acknowledged as a professional.

Traditionally, it was deemed that all professionals wielded considerable power, particularly over nonprofessionals such as the patients, carers, families and other service users. This has changed dramatically, with nonprofessionals now being seen as having more power, particularly in decision-making processes that affect their health and well-being. Further impacted by interprofessional working which is also shifting the balance of power.

Judging professionalism is subjective, but there are guidelines that are shared about how it should be judged:

- Against a set of expectations or standards (NMC)
- From our own personal value set and understanding of what 'professionalism' means
- Maybe situational in nature
- Strongly influenced by culture
- Good health and care outcomes are dependent upon professionalism.

Professionalism is the behaviour that is demonstrated by someone who is a professional in their field which is observed and can be measurable. People also have expectations of what they perceive as professionalism based on the role that is created and understood in the field of practice. It is important as a professional to reflect on one's own behaviour and to think about how others, for example, your clients and coworkers, view your level of professionalism.

Nursing is a self-regulating profession. What this means is that its members establish a set of standards, values, safe practice guidance and ethical frameworks which the professional is expected to adhere to above the minimum standards defined by the law (NMC 2019). Nurses are therefore professionals who have a standardised scope of practice, a professional body for regulation and a professional body of knowledge. For example, nursing has a scope of practice that seeks to create positive change in the lives of people. Thus the NMC code stipulates the professional standards which nurses and midwives must uphold while providing care and when undertaking leadership roles, educating others or conducting research. Therefore, while its values and principles may cover a range of roles and responsibilities and may be subject to interpretation, they are not applied with discretion and are nonnegotiable (NMC 2018).

Professional codes of conduct have clauses which require the individual to consider how conduct in their personal lives influence their profession and that, as such, it is often unanticipated that a professional's personal life is covered within their code of conduct and can impact its reputation (Cornock 2023). Therefore, before we consider the concept of professionalism, we need to consider identity. Identity is an individual's perception of oneself and is as unique and individual as the person. A personal identity is therefore the distinctive characteristics, behaviour, thoughts and emotions of an individual which develop over time (McAdams et al. 2021). Our identities are essential, as they provide our lives with meaning and guidance and impact our behaviour. Personal identity has been a topical debate for many years (Barton and Allan 2015). Traditionally, our identity has been divided into three subdivisions, outlined in Fig. 8.1.

Our identity is determined by our conduct, what we say or write, what other people say about us and through face-to-face interactions.

Conventional wisdom says we should keep our personal and professional lives separate. However, many people actually are beginning to confuse their professional identity with their personal identity, believing that the two of them are completely connected. Although they are not completely separate, there is a need for boundaries.

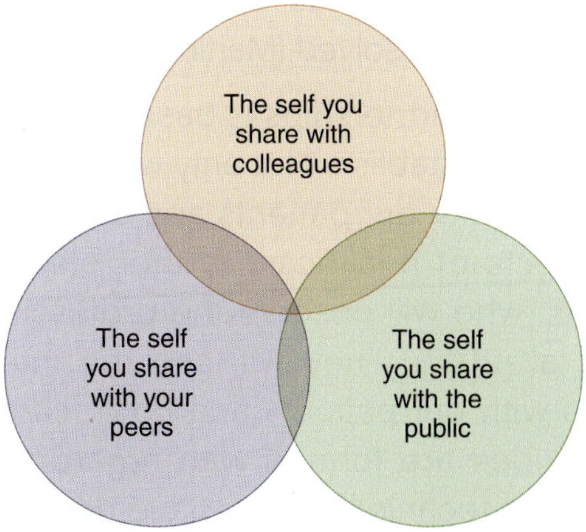

Figure 8.1 Identity subdivisions.

Our personal and professional lives are becoming increasingly fused together due to the power of social media and social networking. This has changed the way we all interact; it is also influencing our personal interests and friends and can have an impact on our professional careers.

The use of social media can provide the outside world with a window into our private lives. Although this can be a positive move in the world of technology, there are some negatives which can impact both one's personal and professional identity (Geraghty et al. 2021). It is therefore important to consider who and what we associate with on social media. For example, acknowledging someone else's post can imply that you endorse or support their point of view. Your patients/clients are not the only people who will be evaluating you as a professional. You will likely be working in teams and with a lot of colleagues who will be judging your professionalism. In addition to this, there is growing interest in the notion of the selfie in the digital age; this type of media type memory brings ethical and moral challenges to the profession. Fundamentally, morals are an individual's internal belief system, whereas ethics are a formalised professional group's system of beliefs of what is right or wrong. As professionals, there is an engagement in a shared belief system which will influence decision making but will also guide displayed behaviour expected of that professional (Cornock 2023). So, while taking a selfie is not forbidden, all professions are built on reputation, and it is important to ensure the professional standard is maintained and that individuals act in a professional manner even when they believe nobody is looking. When behaviour results in the loss of reputation, the public loses trust, and thus the status of a professional within wider society can be dissolved (Martin 2017).

The building of effective partnerships is based on equality; mutual trust and respect take time to establish. Not only will our professional identity impact the relationship with our patients and employers, but one of the most important aspects of healthcare is the role it will play with our juniors and students, who will observe the professional nursing/caring practice (Darch et al. 2017). They will see the interactions between nurses and doctors with our patients and other caring team members Therefore their attitudes are formed with regard to the practice and simultaneous skills and techniques they have observed.

Being a positive role model is an example worthy of being imitated as a professional. Role models of this nature possess qualities that an individual would like to have, and they try to emulate them. Making us want to be better at what we do inspires, motivates and encourages us to try a little harder to be a better nurse, doctor or educator.

What are the individual qualities required to be a role model?

- Passion—Passion for what you do. If you have passion for your job, you are able to inspire others because passion and enthusiasm are contagious. Share your passion. Encourage others to pursue their passions. Lead by example.
- Integrity—Includes such actions as admitting mistakes, being an authentic and genuine person and giving others credit where credit is due, especially in public. It also includes treating people fairly, setting clear values, following through, keeping promises, praising in public and correcting in private, and knowing your limitations. Walk the talk and be humble, as there is always someone smarter, better, faster or more knowledgeable than you.
- Relationship focused—Accepting others as they are, listening to them without judgement and clearly communicating expectations. This includes interacting with others, showing respect for differences and being inclusive rather than exclusive. Individuals who are relationship focused demonstrate concern for others, show a genuine ability to relate to others different from themselves and see the significance and value in others. They also share with others how they make the world a better place.
- Excellence—Demonstrating excellence in your work by being knowledgeable and well rounded, hardworking and pioneering; push the boundaries. Be an early adopter. Employ self-reflection both in general learning and on the impact of your role-modelling efforts.
- Positive choice making—Model positive choice making, think aloud about how you arrived at a solution and explain the rationale behind your decisions.
- Demonstrate confidence—Demonstrating strength and confidence draws admirers. Believe in yourself, believe in others and provide encouragement. Show self-confidence.
- Optimism—Believe that others can grow and change. See the positive in people and give them the benefit of the doubt. If you show that you believe in someone, they will be able to begin to see the possibilities in themselves.

- Resilience/ability to overcome obstacles—Everyone will fail at some time. Everyone will have to overcome obstacles. Learn from your failures. Demonstrate perseverance.
- Generous—Be available and accessible to others and help others as they need. Be generous with your time and attention.
- Community focused—Be involved outside your job and contribute to the community and the profession.

In summary, being a professional is not as simplistic as becoming a member of a professional body postqualification; it encompasses the ability to exercise autonomy; maintain knowledge, skills and ability; and remain committed to the continuity of expected professional behaviour within society, which often can cross the professional and personal boundary.

What are your thoughts on what Sandra Dilks says?

_____
_____
_____
_____
_____

THE ELEMENTS OF PROFESSIONALISM

The words responsibility, integrity, accountability and excellence all spring to mind when thinking about professionalism.

Responsibility—having a strong sense of duty.

Integrity—following values and processes.

Accountability—to accept responsibility for your own actions.

Excellence—to maintain extremely good standards.

8 | NOTES ON WHAT BEING A PROFESSIONAL LOOKS LIKE

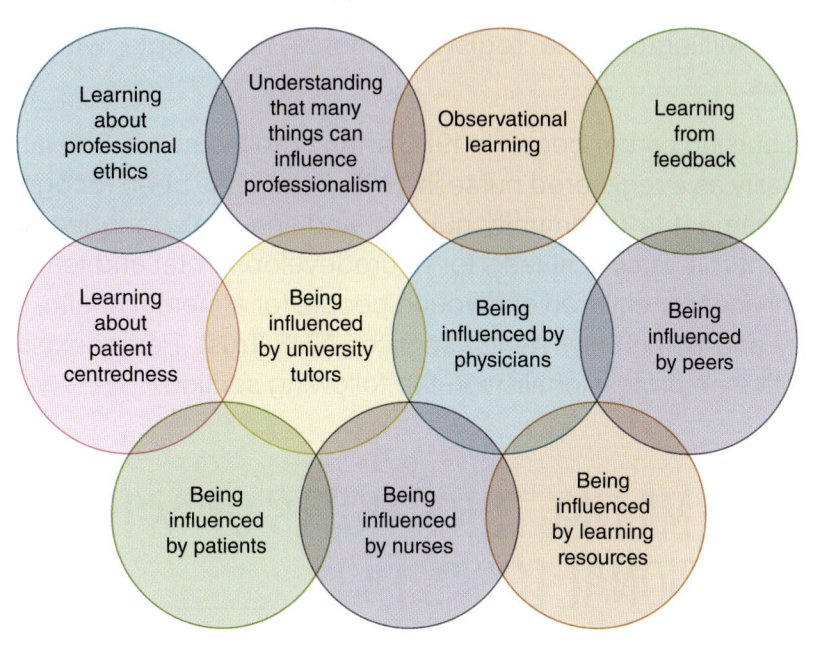

Figure 8.2 12 ways that nursing students develop elements of professionalism in practice.

Without these elements, it will be difficult to maintain and evidence your professionalism. Karimi et al (2014) identify 12 ways that nursing students develop elements of professionalism in their practice. Fig. 8.2 depicts these elements.

> **Think about the elements of professionalism and how and who influences your practice and approach.**
>
> _____
> _____
> _____
> _____
> _____

Penelope Millington is a registered nurse for people with learning disabilities.

Penny's nursing career began in 1985 as an enrolled nurse. She later went on to qualify as a registered nurse in 1990. Penny has been recognised for her commitment to community nursing, and she is also a queen's nurse. Her current role is clinical lead for neurodevelopmental and learning disability services for children and young people for a mental health, learning disability and community health services NHS Trust. Penny explains her perspective on professionalism in the following section.

PENELOPE MILLINGTON'S NOTES ON WHAT BEING A PROFESSIONAL LOOKS LIKE

What does professionalism mean to me as a learning disability nurse? As a learning disability nurse who trained in the 1980s, I have seen first-hand how the profession has changed over the decades. When I started, we wore hats and referred to 'sister' as 'sister'; I still don't know the first names of the sisters from wards 14, 15 and 17. Was this respect or professionalism? Is there a difference? Or is it all one; without respect for others, can we be professional? Is it that the more academic we are, the more we are seen to be professional? Is professionalism also around respect for each other in the nursing and health pathways first and foremost, or is it how others view the nursing profession?

> **THE NMC SAYS**
>
> Promote professionalism and trust:
>
> You uphold the reputation of your profession at all times. You should display a personal commitment to the standards of practice and behaviour set out in the Code. You should be a model of integrity and leadership for others to aspire to. This should lead to trust and confidence in the professions from patients, people receiving care, other health and care professionals and the public.

8 | NOTES ON WHAT BEING A PROFESSIONAL LOOKS LIKE

'Uphold the reputation of your profession at all times'. This statement is something I always remember when I'm out—that I am a nurse, and that this is personally important to me, to ensure that everyone who knows or meets me understands that I am a professional. This has created the person I am today. Every post you make on social media, including photos, the friends that you have on your social media and the posts they make, reflects on you and how you are seen by the outside world.

It is important to remember that the public will judge us by the standards they expect from a nurse.

You should always speak up when you see practice or interactions that are not meeting the standard of care that we should be working towards. Never be afraid to say that you are not happy with a situation that you witness or are involved in. If we do not do this, it is a reflection on us as individuals but also on the profession, and most importantly, it is disrespectful to the patients and their families. They and your colleagues need to be confident that we are providing the best care and interactions possible. Always remember to think—is this okay? Would I be happy with this if it was happening to me or one of my nearest and dearest? If the answer is no, then you need to speak up.

'Lead to trust and confidence in the professions from patients, people receiving care, other health and care professionals and the public'. To me, this statement is about understanding the needs of my service users and their families, never judging or criticising them for the situation that they are in. I aim to be an open book around my involvement and providing care which is person and family centred. While I will listen to all issues, I only offer advice regarding my area of knowledge and within the remit of my role. In addition, I ensure that I am communicating with other agencies to help with areas outside my knowledge and remit and ensure that I am also clear with those agencies with the support I am able to provide. We must never overpromise, as failure to live up to that will end in people feeling that they have been failed by us. Once again, my actions in my personal life, especially when out in public and on social media, need to be considered in light of my profession. What would others think and feel about what I am saying, commenting on or doing?

'Display a personal commitment to the standards of practice and behaviour set out in the Code'. Always remember that you are a nurse first and foremost and that we have a public image. One that needs to be upheld, as we are, and will always be, judged for our career choice.

A thank you from patients and carers is a great compliment; however, the most rewarding thank you is making a difference in a patient's/carer's life. There should be no expectation of gratitude from them; it should be enough that we get a sense of achievement that we have done the role to the best of our ability and made a difference. From delivering bad news to celebrating a recovery or successful change in the quality of life of a patient/carer/family, the knowledge that we have done so with a person-centred approach and have been understanding, responsive and reflective in our actions should be enough.

When considering our interactions with families/patients/carers, it is important to balance the building of rapport against maintaining professionalism. To be able to build a relationship, you need to be skilled and knowledgeable. If you overstep that balance, you risk that professionalism, but if you do not develop the rapport and hide behind being a purely professional nurse, you risk not giving the best evidence-based, person-centred care. So always reflect on your actions and consider how they will be perceived by the patient/family/other carers and the public.

Keeping ourselves up to date within our area of practice will ensure that when working with patients and carers, we show that we are committed to maintaining that high level of understanding, even when that practice is always changing and evolving.

'Be a model of integrity and leadership for others to aspire to'. The next generation of nurses is the most important group of people in our profession. We need to understand the pressures that they are under, but be clear that they have a standard to reach. If these standards are not reached, as nurses, we need to have the courage to advise, support and guide their development. As nurses, we need to continue to maintain our personal and professional development through study and research; this shows others the importance of understanding evidence-based care and therefore providing the most up-to-date care. We cannot say,

'We've always done it like this'; a nurse needs to be able to adapt to new practice from evidence.

We need to show that we are passionate about the role we have and that we are able to motivate others to understand how best to work with a person or other colleagues. If we are not enthusiastic about our role, no one will be, and the profession will lose the respect it has earned from others.

Leadership in the nursing profession is an integral part of the role. We need to ensure that in everything we do, we provide leadership to the colleagues who we come into contact with. This goes further than leading and inspiring our colleagues and other professionals who we come into contact with and includes being able to inspire and lead our patients, families and carers. Failure to provide that leadership could lead to a loss of faith in the profession. As a qualified nurse, being a mentor and ensuring a newly qualified nurse receives a comprehensive preceptorship will ensure that they understand the role and the importance of being part of the nursing profession. It provides support during the changes that happen once you are on the NMC register. A qualified nurse should demonstrate the importance that this has on your life and how you need to behave in all areas and aspects of your everyday living.

In the 1990s, we fought for nursing to be recognised as a profession and not just a vocation; nurses needed to be recognised for their knowledge and skills like teachers and other professionals. A nursing degree was introduced, and we became a workforce with recognised knowledge and skill. Did this change the general public's view, to be seen as a professional group? Within nursing, there has been a battle for recognition, and as learning disability nurses, we may not always have been viewed as 'proper' nurses. In fact, the government did consider stopping the learning disability nurse training. This sometimes places learning disability nurses in a difficult position, and as a professional, I believe that we all need to respect each other's skills and knowledge and be able to reflect on our views and understanding of each group of nursing practitioners.

So, in answer to the questions I posed at the beginning of this piece—as a learning disability nurse, professionalism means that we must always be respectful to everyone that we come into contact with, whether that be in our professional lives or personally. We always need to remember that we are representing our colleagues and the nursing profession at all times. The care that we provide must be evidence based and person centred. We need to be approachable and build rapport with our patients but not overstep the line of professionalism, losing our objectivity around the care we are providing, which will prevent us from delivering the most effective and evidence-based care.

> Write some thoughts about what resonates with you when reading Penelope Millington's perspective on professionalism.
>
> _____
> _____
> _____
> _____

WHAT DOES THIS MEAN IN PRACTICE?

Penelope Millington talks about the NMC code and the section that is entirely focused on professionalism.

> **THE NMC SAYS**
>
> 20 Uphold the reputation of your profession at all times To achieve this, you must:
>
> 20.1 Keep to and uphold the standards and values set out in the Code.
>
> 20.2 Act with honesty and integrity at all times, treating people fairly and without discrimination, bullying or harassment.

20.3 Be aware at all times of how your behaviour can affect and influence the behaviour of other people.

20.4 Keep to the laws of the country in which you are practising.

20.5 Treat people in a way that does not take advantage of their vulnerability or cause them upset or distress.

20.6 Stay objective and have clear professional boundaries at all times with people in your care (including those who have been in your care in the past), their families and carers.

20.7 Make sure you do not express your personal beliefs (including political, religious or moral beliefs) to people in an inappropriate way.

20.8 Act as a role model of professional behaviour for students and newly qualified nurses, midwives and nursing associates to aspire to.

20.9 Maintain the level of health you need to carry out your professional role.

20.10 Use all forms of spoken, written and digital communication (including social media and networking sites) responsibly, respecting the right to privacy of others at all times.

25 Provide leadership to make sure people's well-being is protected and to improve their experiences of the healthcare system.

25.1 Identify priorities, manage time, staff and resources effectively and deal with risk to make sure that the quality of care or service you deliver is maintained and improved, putting the needs of those receiving care or services first, and

25.2 Support any staff you may be responsible for to follow the Code at all times. They must have the knowledge, skills and competence for safe practice; and understand how to raise any concerns linked to any circumstances where the Code has, or could be, broken.

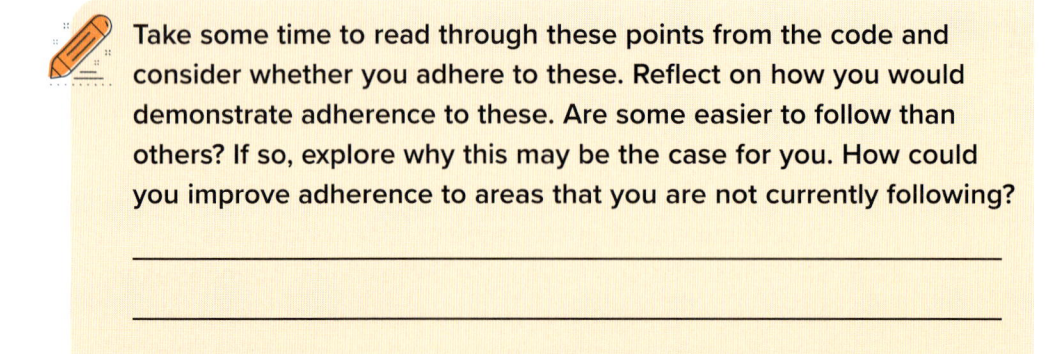

> Take some time to read through these points from the code and consider whether you adhere to these. Reflect on how you would demonstrate adherence to these. Are some easier to follow than others? If so, explore why this may be the case for you. How could you improve adherence to areas that you are not currently following?
>
> _____
> _____
> _____
> _____

It's clear to see that the NMC Code goes some way toward stating what professionalism looks like in practice, but professionalism in practice as a concept is expanded on further in the NMC's 'Enabling professionalism' (NMC 2017) document, which divides professionalism into five distinct headings:

- Learning and developing continuously
- Being a role model for others
- Supporting appropriate service and care environments
- Enabling person-centred and evidence-informed practice
- Leading professionally

Fig. 8.3 depicts how professionalism is defined in the NMC 'Enabling professionalism' document: Robin Binks is a deputy chief nurse at a large acute trust and has been a registered nurse since 2004, spending the majority of his career working with acute providers, with further experience gained at the regional level at NHS Improvement as a clinical advisor. He joined University Hospitals of Leicester (UHL) in August 2022 as deputy chief nurse. Prior to this, he has held several senior leadership roles, including interim chief nurse, deputy chief nurse and head of nursing. Robin explores the concept of what professionalism

8 | NOTES ON WHAT BEING A PROFESSIONAL LOOKS LIKE

Leading professionally by:
- Seeking connection to and support from professional bodies and organisations
- Developing self to lead strategically
- Developing others to lead strategically
- Supporting those in leadership SMART ART

Enabling person-centred and evidence-informed practice by:
- Incorporating up-to-date evidence in daily practice
- Sharing and disseminating evidence-informed practice
- Participation in the generation of new evidence and working innovatively
- Lobbying for change and improvement

Supporting appropriate service and care environments by:
- Raising concerns when issues arise that could compromise safety, quality and experience
- Supporting others to raise concerns appropriately
- Defining and understanding clear referral pathways to support standards of professional practice
- Delegate tasks and duties safely
- Identifying appropriate professional support networks for self and others
- Working collegiately with other professions

Being a role model for others by
- Demonstrating and articulating clearly what professionalism looks like in practice
- Demonstrating positive behaviours and attitudes towards diversity
- Working within a clear professional career framework
- Supporting colleagues and students
- Celebrating personal success and that of others
- Developing people to take on senior roles and supporting those in senior roles
- Treating others with a positive regard
- Providing meaningful and constructive feedback to others

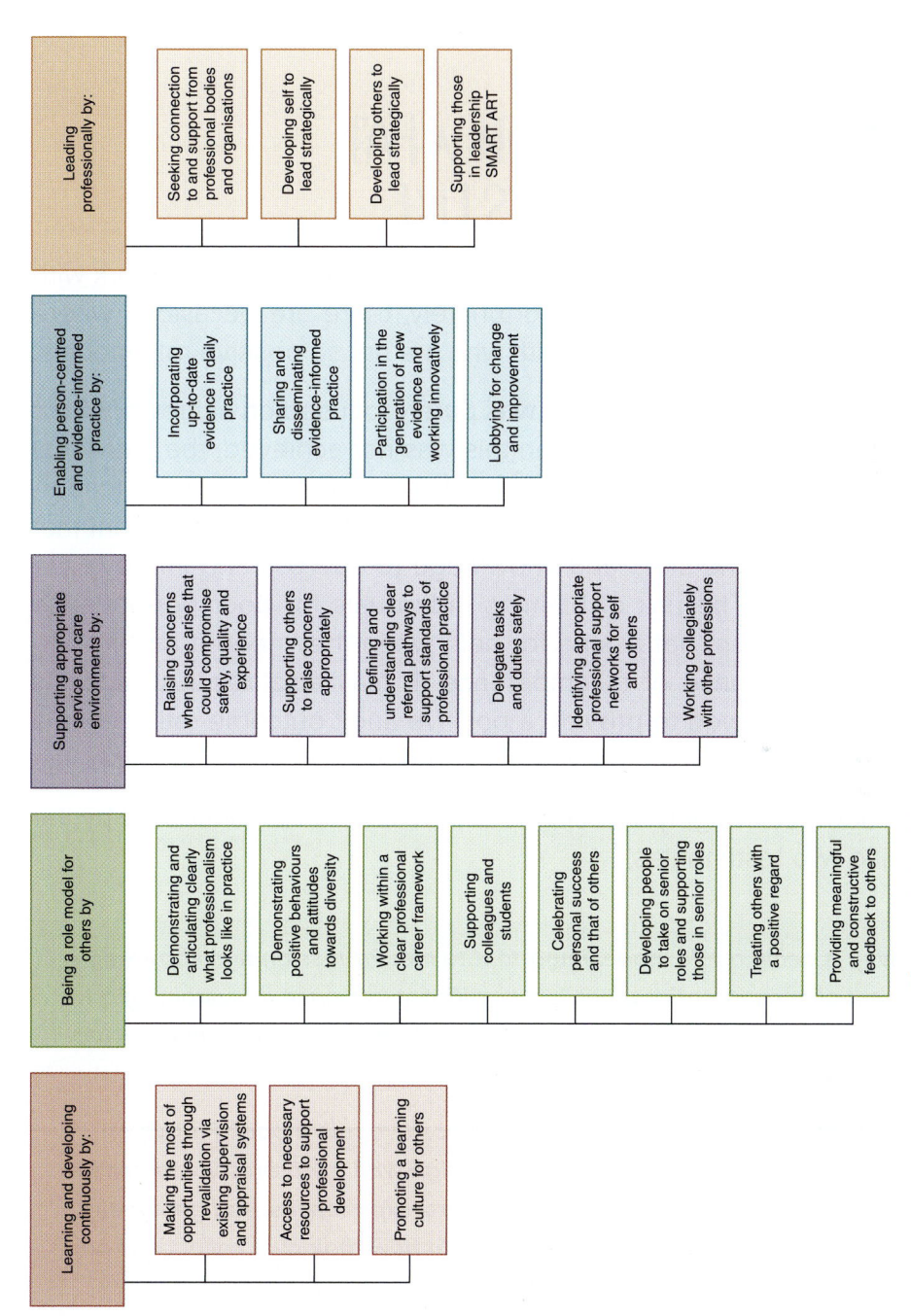

Learning and developing continuously by:
- Making the most of opportunities through revalidation via existing supervision and appraisal systems
- Access to necessary resources to support professional development
- Promoting a learning culture for others

Figure 8.3 How the NMC define professionalism.

means for further practice when explaining what professionalism means to him as follows:

ROBIN BINKS'S NOTES ON WHAT PROFESSIONALISM LOOKS LIKE

Throughout our careers as nurses, many of us are fortunate to work with some excellent role models; unfortunately, there are occasions where there are people who we work with who are not so positive role models.

One person springs to mind who was purely focused on achieving 100% across all quality audits, and when this was not achieved, the individual would vocalise their disappointment and state it was due to poor leadership. The delivery of high-quality care is essential, but it is important that colleagues have the skills and knowledge to address and improve the care we deliver. The risk of blaming individuals for poor performance could result in them not asking for help when they need it and feeling isolated and a sense of incompetence. It may also result in specific items being reviewed to provide a positive audit outcome rather than a transparent review, which provides a true reflection of the situation.

Role models can hugely influence our practice, as demonstrated by the following two testimonies.

> 'Why is being a role model important to me: Professional acknowledgment of my authentic values is a significant influence in sustaining a genuine connection with colleagues and is one of the fundamental reasons I enjoy my senior leadership role in nursing.
>
> How do I benefit from others being a positive role model: I thrive on surrounding myself with people who align with my professional belief system. I also enjoy learning from others' experiences, so I genuinely appreciate when people are open about how their own reflections have served them in continual learning'.
>
> **Sue Chisholm, divisional nurse at Nottingham University Hospitals**

8 | NOTES ON WHAT BEING A PROFESSIONAL LOOKS LIKE

> '*Why is being a role model important to me:* The benefits of being a positive role model are twofold. Being able to guide, support and coach someone to being their best self and knowing, due to your role as a leader, there are excellent role models for the next generation. I thrive on engaging and developing others to reach their full potential; it is the best part of being a senior leader.
>
> *How do I benefit from others being a positive role model:* In a world driven by social media and sharing all that's good in people's lives, I find it more important than ever to have authentic leaders. Role models who are humble, honest and willing to show their flaws and challenges. Enabling others to share how they have learned from their mistakes and challenges to drive change and make a real difference'.
>
> **Belinda Dring, divisional nurse at Nottingham University Hospitals**

Whether you are a new or experienced registrant, we are, as a team, collectively responsible for creating a healthy workplace that attracts and retains the best members (Cummings et al. 2010). This can be achieved by us all being effective role models. Murray and Main (2005) describe role modelling as a process that allows individuals to learn new behaviours and skills through a structured process of observing and learning instead of via a process of trial and error. Dake and Taylor (1994) describe role modelling as 'teaching by example and learning by imitation'; the nature of nursing means role modelling is fundamental to professional socialisation (Lynn 1995). When role models are effective, this creates an environment where individuals want to acquire new skills and do their best when they feel free to express and choose their own direction (Murray and Main 2005). As an expert or novice registrant within the workplace, we are role models by default, as every action we take and how we deal with a situation are observed by colleagues, patients or members of the public, and in the future, this behaviour may influence others' behaviour and experiences (Shirey 2006). The mood and behaviour we display creates a lasting impression on those around use (Porter-O'Grady 2003). As a profession, we are all contributors to excellence in practice, colleague engagement and patient satisfaction, and we are collectively responsible for creating and supporting an environment where we can develop as clinical experts and future healthcare leaders (Espionoza et al. 2009). As healthcare providers, we are in a public-facing role and are often viewed by patients and members of the public and nonclinical colleagues as the face of the organisation that links organisations directly with their experience, which, in turn, can have a direct impact on quality of care, experience and satisfaction of service users when accessing our services (Lucas et al. 2008, Shirey 2006). Appointing the right team members is essential, as they can have a direct impact on the quality of care delivered to patients and colleagues (Shirey 2006). As role models and individual practitioners, we can influence the working environments by decreasing stress and increasing communication, job satisfaction and patient safety (Shirey 2006). Without knowing and irrespective of being an expert or novice, we all provide support and guidance to those around us (Squires 2004).

As registered practitioners having an understanding and collective awareness of the complexities of the environment we work within, and embracing our position as role models, we can translate and deliver change in a meaningful and sustainable way for colleagues and service users (Malloch and Porter-O'Grady 2009). If this is done in a negative way, it can have an adverse effect on the team we are working with, which can be detrimental to service delivery and patient outcomes. By contributing to the development of a positive environment that will, in turn, allow a culture of autonomy in appropriate decision making, participation in unit and hospital governance and participative management may be the best strategies for retaining colleagues in the hospital setting and creating a better place to work (Gormley 2011).

Leveck and Jones (1996) state that the culture within the team contributes mostly to retention and quality of the team. Our leadership behaviour has been directly attributed to being a primary factor that is most likely to improve job satisfaction and retention of our colleagues (Andrews and Dziegielewski 2005). The more visible and positive role model we are within the unit/ward, that is, not delivering care from behind the nurses' station, the more colleagues will perceive us as being more involved and caring about how the shift and the quality of care that is delivered to patients (Feather et al. 2015). Visibility needs to be meaningful and serve a purpose; just because we are seen in practice does not mean we are being proactive and effective.

Within the ward/unit environment, we often look to those around us in more senior roles, specifically the ward/unit manager to guide us and be our sole role models. Unfortunately, there is varied consideration that it is difficult for the ward/unit manager to be visible 365 days a year, 24 hours a day when the majority are single post holders and contracted to work 37.5 hours per week, which equates to 22.3% of the time (excluding annual leave). With rota schedules covering 24 hours per day, the ward manager can go for periods of time without seeing their team simply because of opposite shift patterns. Taking this into consideration, it really highlights the importance we all have as leaders and in being the best role model but also the importance of our leadership, whether we are an expert or novice practitioner.

The literature identifies that our roles are forever changing, increasingly challenging and often demanding. Sometimes with the negative media coverage, it is a difficult balance to get right. However, collectively, we need to empower each other as members of the workforce, ensuring where appropriate that we involve ourselves in the decision-making process of the unit/team/organisation and, if possible, provide supportive guidance without being the worst version of ourselves. For some of our current and future colleagues, not maintaining a balanced approach/keeping it real may contribute to an unrealistic view of the role. This may result in further recruitment and retention issues. We need to remain balanced in our roles, both sharing the positives and negatives, so those around us truly understand and have awareness of the challenges and situations we face. If we get the balance right in practice, then future post holders would be aware of every element of the role and have the skills to address them (Titzer et al. 2013).

The responsibility of being effective role models should be an organisational priority and not solely senior colleagues' responsibility. Darbyshire (2010) identified where colleagues described a culture that verbal abuse and disrespect among colleagues were commonplace; this had a direct correlation with staff satisfaction and, in turn, recruitment and retention. In organisations where everyone acts as a role model, better retention of staff has been observed (Pfeffer 2007).

> **TIPS**
>
> Professionalism can seem like quite an abstract concept, so it's a good idea to reflect on your own professionalism by asking a few questions:
>
> Consider:
>
> - Do your colleagues always see the best version of you?
> - Are you always the best role model you can be?
>
> Think who your role models are.
>
> - What makes them a good role model?
> - What have you learnt from them?
> - How have they shaped your style?
>
> Always take time to reflect on the negative role models you have encountered.
>
> - What made it a negative experience?
> - What did you learn from them?
> - What would you do differently?

We can all impact on-the-job satisfaction of colleagues without knowing, and therefore without being aware, that we are role models, and the impact our behaviour has on others is not preparing us for current roles or future roles (Collins and Collins 2007).

CARING WITH CONFIDENCE: THE CODE IN ACTION

In 2020, the NMC launched some animated resources for the code to help registrants have confidence in their decisions and actions: 'Caring With Confidence: The Code in Action' (NMC 2020). Each video is under 3 minutes long, and the topics they explore are:

- Accountability
- Professional judgement

- Delegation
- Speaking up
- Being inclusive and challenging discrimination
- Social media
- Person-centred care
- End-of-life care
- Professionalism

These animations demonstrate that to keep people's trust, you need to live up to the expectations that others have. It highlights how professionalism goes hand in hand with leadership. They define leadership as being a role model, influencing future generations. It does not mean that you must have a formal leadership job role, as the NMC recognises that all nursing roles will have opportunities to utilise leadership qualities throughout day-to-day practice. There are ways that you can have influence by considering the role you play within a team and the dynamics of the team, being aware of your own strengths and weaker areas, recognising strengths and weaknesses in others, and supporting others who are doing the right thing. These are all elements of leadership qualities that you can utilise from the start of your career.

Dedication and commitment are required to maintain the trust and confidence that others have in you. Continually striving to improve your practice and develop yourself as a nurse is a way to demonstrate this. This can be achieved by regular reflections on your practice, engaging in learning opportunities and seeking feedback from colleagues and patients.

PROFESSIONALISM IN A WIDER CONTEXT

So far in this chapter, we have looked at many different aspects of what professionalism is, but how does this differ from other occupations and nationalities? And importantly, how is it attracting and retaining both domestically and internationally educated nurses during a time of crisis within the nursing workforce?

Heidi Dine is the lead nurse for the United Kingdom's largest supplier of international educated nurses to the National Health Service and talks about the wider global perspective:

HEIDI DINE'S NOTES ON WHAT PROFESSIONALISM LOOKS LIKE

I am often told by our new recruits of their excitement of joining the 'UK's nursing profession'.

> 'The UK has the most prestigious nursing profession in the world. There is such a long history of nursing development in England, starting with Florence Nightingale, through to the large historic hospitals and, of course, the NHS, which employs more nurses than any other healthcare provider. I can't wait to see where I can take my career!'
>
> **Alina, adult nurse educated in India**

The notion of nursing as a profession is one that has been deliberated and debated for many years, and yet still there is no consensus as to what exactly a 'professional nurse' is. The concept of 'professionalism' itself is complex and multidimensional and varies over time, countries and cultures, attitudes and activities. However, professionalism is consistently noted as having a positive impact on nursing and increasing care quality, patient safety and staff autonomy (Cao et al. 2023). It can also have a positive influence on an individual's job satisfaction, career aspirations and length of service. It is therefore vital that all nurses understand the complexities of belonging to a profession and are able to draw upon the benefits of this into their daily practice and interaction with patients.

THE NMC SAYS

Promote professionalism and trust

You uphold the reputation of your profession at all times. You should display a personal commitment to the standards of practice and behaviour set out in the Code. You should be a model of integrity and leadership for others to aspire to. This should lead to trust and confidence in the professions from patients, people receiving care, other health and care professionals and the public.

The history of nursing as a profession

The Cambridge Dictionary Definition of 'profession' includes a 'type of job that is respected because it involves a high level of education and training'.

(Cambridge University press) and, interestingly, the example given include that of a nurse. However, the traditional view of the nursing profession was far removed from this explanation. Nursing was historically seen as a 'calling profession' (Kallio et al 2022), perhaps a remnant of when many nursing staff members were also religious sisters. Throughout the history of nursing, the profession and those involved have travelled through various incarnations of public images—the caring angel, the doctor's handmaiden, the battleaxe stern authority of the 1950s, quickly followed by the 'naughty nurses' in *Carry On Matron* (Gonzalez et al. 2023) and the 'superheroes' who were clapped and revered through the COVID pandemic. The professionalisation of nurses through education and advances has largely taken place in the background of media clichés, and as a result, the expansion of the nurse's role and the growth in the status of the professional is sadly still not yet recognised by the majority of the wider public (ten Hoeve et al. 2014)

> *'I was talking to my dad's friend about the nursing strikes. He commented that he didn't understand why nurses needed a degree "to wipe bums". While I was shocked by his comment, I also realised that he had an outdated view which needed addressing. I explained that in my role as an advanced nurse practitioner that I needed to have not just a BSc but an MSc. I spoke to him about my work as an independent autonomous practitioner. By the end of the conversation, he said that he didn't realise the additional roles of nurses, and I was pleased I was able to educate him'.*
>
> **Louise, advanced nurse practitioner**

The Royal College of Nursing (RCN) has recently updated its definition of nursing, stating that an update was required due to demonstrate the 'safety-critical role and increased complexity' of nursing (RCN 2023) and notes that more needs to be done to ensure that the public is aware of the growing dimensions of nursing.

Professional identity

Professional identity is how we define ourselves by the work that we do. It is a component of our complete identity and includes how we feel are seen by society and how the public interacts with them and how we interpret these encounters (Sutherland et al. 2010). Therefore, although it is an individual and personal concept, it is inextricably linked to external influence. Indeed, it can often be present before a nurse even enters the profession (Lyneham and Levett-Jones 2016).

> 'When I was 7, I had to have my appendix out. I don't remember much about it, but I do know that's when I made the decision to become a nurse. The nurses on the ward were all so lovely and made me feel safe and cared for. When I started on the wards for the first time, I wanted to care for my patients in the way that I was cared for'.
>
> *Teresa, children's nurse*

It can therefore be argued that it is essential that the concept of professionalism and professional identity is taught to undergraduate nurses throughout their nurse training and that active discussion around the concept of professional identity helps to develop established and invested nurses (Fitzgerald and Cluckey 2020). In order to fully adopt the role of a nurse, it is essential that students' education results in them *'thinking, acting and feeling like a Nurse'* (Godfrey and Young 2021, p. 363). I feel it is very reminiscent of the famous Florence Nightingale quote that a nurse should use her 'brain, heart and hands', perhaps suggesting that, in fact, the basics of nursing professionalism have changed very little in over a century. Liebig and Embree (2023) suggest that educators use four key domains to support nurses' professionalism education: values and ethics, knowledge, the nurse as a leader and professional comportment.

8 | NOTES ON WHAT BEING A PROFESSIONAL LOOKS LIKE

Comportment refers to a nurse's professional behaviour as demonstrated through actions and interactions and therefore is a fundamental 'building block' upon which to develop a student's ability to cooperate, connect and relate to both the team in which they work and the patients they care for. Clinker and Shirley (2013) go further and urge that the dimension of comportment is as important to developing nursing practice as the advancement of clinical practices. In their research, they devise a comprehensive approach to the development comportment for nurses by the integration of key professional fundamentals:

Fig. 8.4

Antecedents
- Capacity for compassion
- Confidence
- Emotional intelligence
- Human dignity
- Reflection
- Regulation
- Self-awareness
- Values and beliefs

Theoretical definition: A nurse's professional behaviour that integrates value, virtues and mores through words, actions, presence and deeds.

Operational definition: A nurse's set of defining behaviours that integrates consistently between values and actions and may be measured in the form of professional conduct, appearance and collaborative practice.

Critical attributes
- Mutual respect
- Beliefs and actions are harmonious and consistent
- Commitment
- Collaboration

Professional comportment

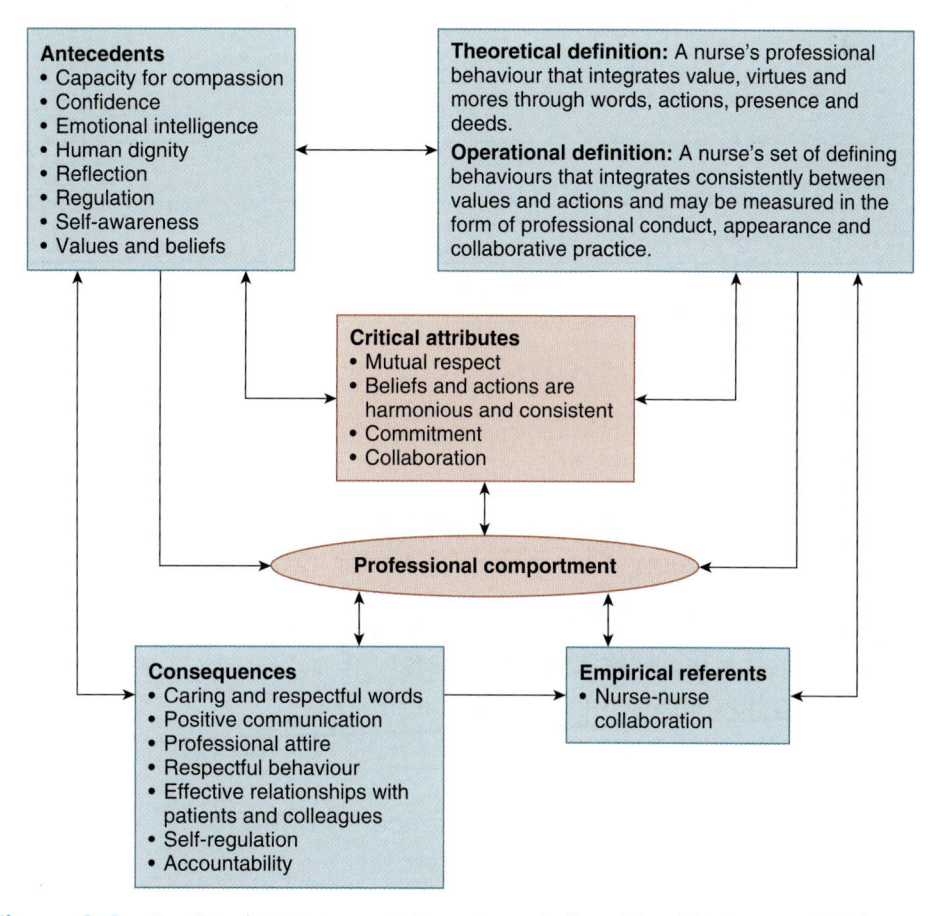

Consequences
- Caring and respectful words
- Positive communication
- Professional attire
- Respectful behaviour
- Effective relationships with patients and colleagues
- Self-regulation
- Accountability

Empirical referents
- Nurse-nurse collaboration

Figure 8.4   Professional comportment as defined by Clinker and Shirley (2013).

The use of models and criteria to define nursing as a profession is not a new concept. Miller et al. (1993) created the '9 standards criteria for the nursing profession': educational background, adherence to the code of ethics, participation in professional organisations, continuing education and competency, communication and publication, autonomy and self-regulation, community service, and research and theory. This may seem like a long list of requirements; however, they are very closely linked to the professional standards expected from the NMC.

> Think about each of these components, review the NMC code and cross reference. How do they match up?
>
> _____
> _____
> _____
> _____
> _____

There are numerous further examples of concepts and models of the nursing profession. For example, Yoder (2017) believed nursing professionalism had six core concepts:

1. Acting in the patient's best interests
2. Showing humanism
3. Practising social responsibility
4. Demonstrating sensitivity
5. Having high standards of competence/knowledge
6. Demonstrating high ethical standards.

These varying opinions among academics further demonstrate the multifaceted and complexity of nurses' identities.

8 | NOTES ON WHAT BEING A PROFESSIONAL LOOKS LIKE

While it is perhaps inevitable that external forces have an impact upon how the nursing profession views itself, it is perhaps more important for nurses to consider how they view and portray themselves professionally. What is the nurse's own sense of professional identity? The need for an internal validation and collective agreement is paramount if nurses are to promote the nursing profession; however, research shows that this is often lacking in many nursing colleagues (Rozani et al 2023). Without a consensus of what it means to be a professional, nurses will struggle to identify the attributes within themselves and others that shape their work and, in turn, will be unable to quantify these attributes when advocating and promoting the profession, directly impacting recruitment and retention.

> *'When I first gave up my clinical nursing role and moved into one based in quality (more office based), it did take me some time to adjust, both personally and professionally. I found it difficult to explain and justify my role. Now that I have worked in this role for some time, I feel my more confident about my own identity. I think that this was a process I had to go through, but by always relating my work back to the (NMC) Code and the patient, I feel that I am still very much "a nurse"'.*
>
> **Katy, quality and improvement senior nurse**

Personal reflection

Nurses with a strong professional identity are those who stand out among nursing colleagues, and as a nursing student, I remember Nurse Miriam fondly. She embodied my image of nursing—caring, experienced, calm and educated. Nothing seemed to fluster her. And her passion for her work was infectious. I wanted to become a nurse just like her!

I have been qualified as a nurse for almost 25 years now. During this time, I have worked in a variety of positions within acute and nonscheduled care, in the community, within the NHS, for private companies and now for NHS professionals. I have moved from very clinical roles into managerial and strategic positions with no clinical work. However, throughout all these transitions, I have always continued to view myself as 'a nurse' and have always been very proud of this fact. Within society and the profession, there is a more traditional view of 'the bedside nurse'; however, changes to the way nursing is taught and the many differing roles and careers that nursing can lead to are helping to change the lens through which people see nurses and how we view ourselves.

> 'I think that, moving forward, the notion and identity of what it is to be a nurse will change. I do not think that the notion of nurses taking on additional responsibilities, working in corporate or nonclinical roles, or moving away from the bedside will be seen as "unusual". Indeed, I think that moving forward, we will see more opportunities for nurses to expand their roles'.
>
> *Nathan, senior nurse*

Think about your own experiences. Which nurse has stood out to you and why?

_____
_____
_____
_____
_____

Teaching and developing professionalism

As one would imagine, with an issue as complex as this, opinions on how to teach professionalism and develop a culture of professional proficiency are varied. Role modelling is noted as a key component in helping to establish a culture of professionalism (Fitzgerald and Clukey

2020). However, poor conditions and professional examples can do as much or more damage than positive ones. We know that constructive environments and atmospheres can help to shape and improve student nurses' professional identities and, alongside, increase retention (Zeng et al. 2022)

Global perspective

The World Health Organization (WHO) informs that there are 28 million nurses working across the world, which represents 59% of the total number of all health professionals (WHO 2020). Internationally, 86% of countries regulate nurses via the use of a governing body; however, regulation of both training and standards is not consistent, and the WHO urges that 'professional nursing regulation must be modernized', citing a need for regulatory frameworks, scopes of practice and education and credentialing standards. This therefore can lead to varying opinions globally on nurses' professionalism.

Despite the various types of training, career opportunities and scope of practice, almost universally, nurses are seen as trusted and caring individuals and are known to centre the care that they give around the patient. They are a respected professional and often held with high moral regard (Ulrich 2021). What can vary is the degree to which nurses are seen as autonomous practitioners in their own right and therefore the level to which they are able to assert their knowledge and strive to improve and reflect upon care. These are values that are at the very heart of the NMC code and of every professional nurse working in the United Kingdom.

CONCLUSION

Professionalism is an essential part of being a nurse and an integral part of adhering to the NMC code of conduct. Consistently demonstrating professional behaviour will help you to develop your professional relationships with patients and colleagues alike and ensure you flourish as a nurse. Not only are you responsible for your own professionalism, but you also have a responsibility to speak out when others are not following this.

Remember, reflective practice will help you to check in with your professional conduct and consider areas for further improvement. Being able to openly reflect and continually grow and learn will also help with evidencing how you are adhering to the code of conduct for your ongoing revalidation. The earlier you can start reflecting and linking your practice to the code, the easier this process will become for you. Remember that professionalism is your personal responsibility.

Space for reader's own reflection:

REFERENCES

Andrews, D.R., Dziegiewski, S.F., 2005. The nurse manager: Job satisfaction, the nurse shortage and retention. J. Nurs. Manag 13, 286−295.

Barton, T., Allan, D., 2015. Advanced Nursing Practice: Changing healthcare in a changing world. Palgrave, London.

Cambridge Dictionary. 2023. Cambridge Dictionary. https://dictionary.cambridge.org/dictionary/english/professional [Accessed January 18, 2024]

Cambridge University Press. n.d. Profession. In Cambridge Dictionary. https://dictionary.cambridge.org/dictionary/english/profession [Accessed August 3, 2024]

Cao, H., Song, Y., Wu, Y., He, X., Chen, Y., Wang, Q., et al., 2023. What is nursing professionalism? A concept analysis. BMC Nurs 22 (34), 1−14.

Clinker, D.A., Shirley, M., 2013. Professional comportment: The missing element in nursing practice. Nurs. Forum 48 (2) 106−113.

Collins, S.K., Collins, K.S., 2007. Changing workforce demographics necessitates succession planning in healthcare. Health Care Manag 26 (4).

Cornock, M., 2023. Accountability and Professionalism in Nursing and Healthcare. London, Sage.

Cummings, G., MacGregor, T., Davey, M., Lee, H., Wong, C., Muise, M., et al., 2010. Leadership styles and outcome patterns for the nursing workforce and work environment: A systematic review. International journal of nursing studies 47 (3), 363–385.

Dake, S.B., Taylor, J.A. 1994. Do as I do: The importance of the clinical instructor as role model. J. Extra Corpor. Technol 26 (3), 140−142.

Darbyshire, P., 2010. Wonderful workplace or woeful workhouse? Start creating a more positive workplace culture today. Contemp. Nurse 36 (1−2).

Darch, J., Baillie, L., Gillison, F., 2017. Nurses as role models in health promotion: A concept analysis. Br. J. Nurs 26 (17), 982–988.

Espionoza, D.C., Lopez-Saldana, A., Stonestreet, J.S., 2009. The pivotal role of the nurse manager in healthy workplaces. Crit. Care Nurs. Q 32 (4), 327−334.

Feather, R.A., Ebright, P., Bakas, T., 2015. Nurse Manager behaviours that RNs perceive to affect their job satisfaction. Nurs. Forum. Wiley Periodicals.

Fitzgerald, A., Clukey, L., 2020. Professional identity in graduating nursing students. J. Nurs. Educ 60 (2), 74−80.

Geraghty, S., Hari, R., Oliver, K., 2021. Using social media in contemporary nursing: Risks and benefits. Br. J. Nurs 30 (18), 1078–1082.

Godfrey, N., Young, E., 2021. Professional Identity. In: Giddends, J. (Ed.), Concepts of Nursing Practice, third ed. Elsevier.

Gonzalez, H., Errasti-Ibarrondo, B., Iraizoz-Iraizoz, A., Choperena, A., 2023. The image of nursing in the media: A scoping review. Int. Nurs. Rev 70, 425−443.

Gormley, D., 2011. Are we on the same page? Staff nurse and manager preceptions of work environment, quality of care and anticipated nurse turnover. J. Nurs. Manag 19, 33−40.

Ipsos. 2018. Ipsos MORI Veracity Index. https://www.ipsos.com/sites/default/files/ct/news/documents/2018-11/veracity_index_2018_v1_161118_public.pdf [Accessed October 20, 2023]

Kallio, H., Kangesniemi, M., Hult, M., 2022. Registered nurses' perceptions of their career-An interview study. J. Nurs. Manag 30, 3378−3385.

Karimi, Z., Ashktorab, T., Mohammadi, E., Abedi, H.A., 2014. Using the hidden curriculum to teach professionalism in nursing students. Iran. Red Crescent Med. J 16 (3).

Liebig, D., Embree, J., 2023. Teaching Professional Compartment. J. Contin. Educ. Nurs 54 (5), 204−207.

Leveck, M.L., Jones, C.B., 1996. The Nursing Practice environment, staff retention, and quality of care. Res. Nurs. Health 19 (4), 331−343.

Lucas, V., Laschinger, H., Wong, C., 2008. The impact of emotional intelligent leadership on staff nurse empowerment: The moderating effect of span of control. J. Nurs. Manag.

Lyneham, J., Levett-Jones, T., 2016. Insights into registered nurses' professional values through the eyes of graduating students. Nurse Educ. Pract 17, 86–90. https://doi. org/10.1016/j.nepr.2015.11.002

Lynn, M.R., 1995. Development and testing of the nursing role model competence scale. J. Nurs. Meas 3, 2.

Malloch, K., Porter-O'Grady, T., 2009. The quantum leader: Applications for the new world of work. Jones and Bartlett Publishers.

Martin, L., 2017. Professionalism: In the eye of the beholder. Paediatr. Anaesth 27 (3), 226−227.

McAdams, D., Trzesniewski, K., Lilgendahl, J., Benet-Martonez, V., Robins, R., 2021. Self and Identity in Personality Psychology. Personality Science. https://ps.psychopen.eu/index.php/ps/article/view/6035/6035.html [Accessed September 27, 2023]

Miller, B.K., Adams, D., Bark, L., 1993. A behavioural inventory for professionalism in nursing. J. Prof. Nurs 9 (5), 290–295.

Murray, C., Main, A., 2005. Role modelling as a teaching method for student mentors. Nurs. Times 101, 26.

Nursing and Midwifery Council. 2017. Enabling professionalism in nursing and midwifery practice. https://www.nmc.org.uk/globalassets/sitedocuments/other-publications/enabling-professionalism.pdf [Accessed January 7, 2025]

Nursing and Midwifery Council. 2018. The Code Professional Standards of Practice and Behaviour for Nurses and Midwives Nursing and Midwifery Council [Online]. Nursing and Midwifery Council. London, Nursing and Midwifery Council, p.10. https://www.nmc.org.uk/globalassets/sitedocuments/nmc-publications/nc-code.pdf.

Nursing and Midwifery Council. 2019. Legislative requirement for regulating education standards. https://www.nmc.org.uk/education/our-role-in-education/legislative-requirement-for-regulating-education-standards/ [Accessed September 27, 2023]

Nursing and Midwifery Council. 2020. Caring with Confidence: The Code in Action [Online]. https://www.nmc.org.uk/standards/code/code-in-action/ [Accessed January 18, 2024]

Oxford Learners Dictionary. n.d. Professionalism noun − Definition, pictures, pronunciation and usage notes /Oxford Advanced Learner's Dictionary. OxfordlLearnersDictionaires.com [online] https://www.oxfordlearnersdictionaries.com/definition/english/professionalism. [Accessed January 18, 2024]

Pfeffer, J., 2007. Human resources from an organisational behaviour perspective: Some paradoxes explained. J. Econ. Perspect 21 (4), 115–134.

Porter-O'Grady, T., 2003. A Different Age for Leadership, part 2: New Rules, New Roles. J. Nurs. Adm 33 (3), 173–178.

Rozani, V., Kagan, I., 2023. Factors associated with the extent of nurses' involvement in the promotion of the nursing profession: A cross-sectional study among nurses working in diverse healthcare settings. BMC Nurs 23 (49), 1–8.

Royal College of Nursing. 2023. New Definition of Nursing captures Profession's Complexity, https://rcni.com/nursing-standard/newsroom/news/new-definition-of-nursing-captures-professions-complexity-200421 [Accessed January 18, 2024]

Shirey, M.R., 2006. Stress and coping in nurse managers: Two decades of research. Nurs. Econ 24 (4), 193–203.

Squires, A., 2004. A dimensional analysis of role enactment of acute care nurses. J. Nurs. Sch 36 (3), 272–278.

Sutherland, L., Howard, S., Markauskaite, L., 2010. Professional identity creation: Examining the development of preservice teachers' under-standing of their work as teachers. Teach. Teach. Educ 263, 455–465.

ten Hoeve, Y., Jansen, G., Roodbol, P., 2014. The nursing profession: public image, self concept and professional identity: A discussion paper. J. Adv. Nurs 70 (2), 295–309.

Titzer, J., Phillips, T., Tooley, S., Hall, N., Shirey, M., 2013. Nurse Manager Succession planning: Synthesis of the evidence. J. Nurs. Manag 21 (7), 971–979.

Ulrich, B., 2021. Imagine a world without nurses – Understanding our value and worth and upholding the standards of our profession. Nephrol. Nurs. J 48 (6), 523. https://doi.org/10.37526/1526-744X.2021.48. 6.523

World Health Organisation. 2020. State of the World's Nursing: Executive Summary [Online]. https://iris.who.int/bitstream/handle/10665/331673/9789240003293-eng.pdf [Accessed January 18, 2024]

Yoder, L., 2017. Professionalism in nursing. MedSurg Nurs 26(5), 293–295.

Zeng, L., Chen, Q., Fan, S., Yi, Q., An, W., Liu, H., et al., 2022. Factors influencing the professional identity of nursing interns: a cross-sectional study. BMC Nurs. 21 (1), 200. https://bmcnurs.biomedcentral.com/articles/10.1186/s12912-022-00983-2 [Accessed February 3, 2025]

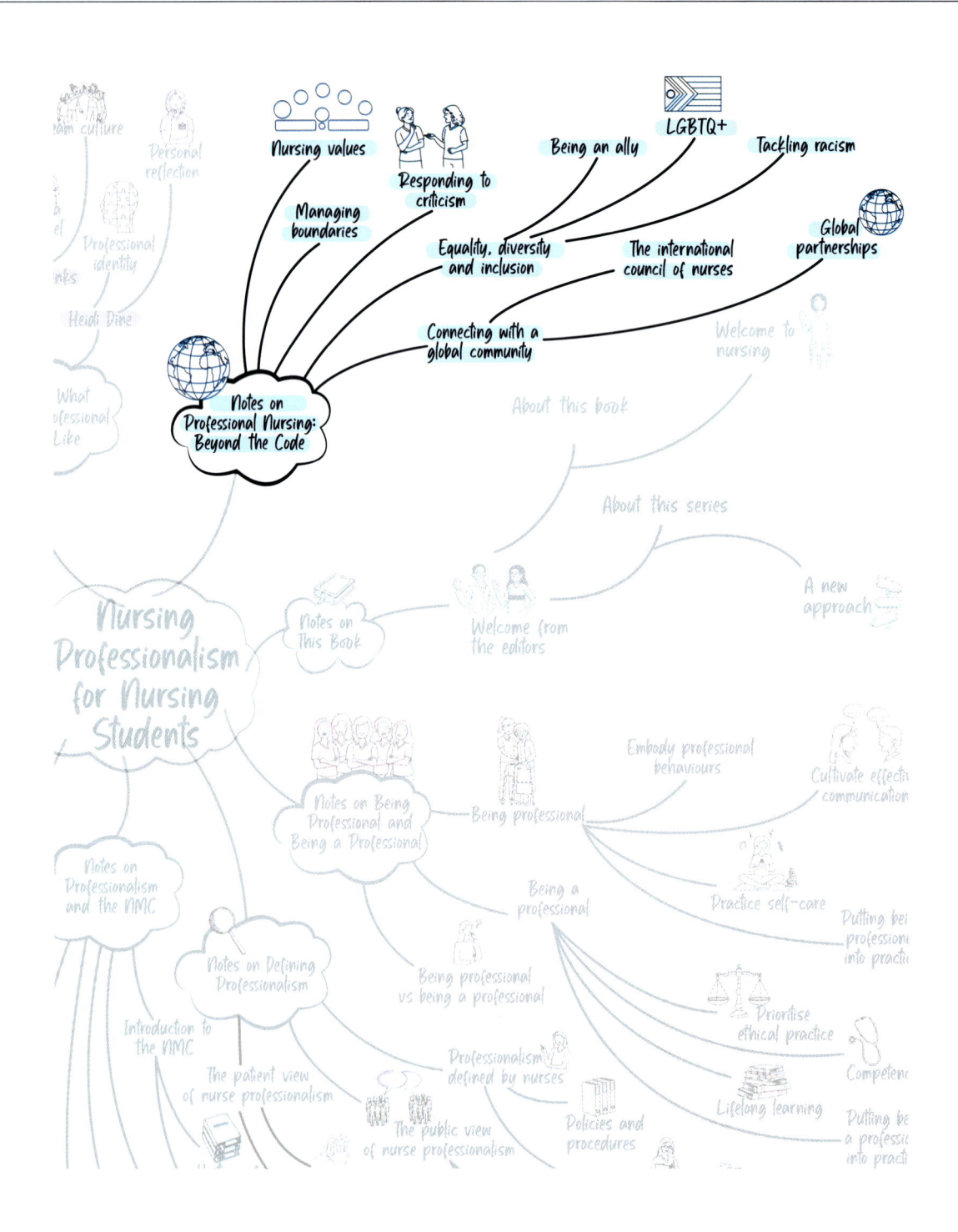

Notes on Professional Nursing: Beyond the Code

- Nursing values
- Responding to criticism
- Managing boundaries
- Being an ally
- LGBTQ+
- Tackling racism
- Equality, diversity and inclusion
- The international council of nurses
- Global partnerships
- Connecting with a global community

9

NOTES ON PROFESSIONAL NURSING: BEYOND THE CODE

Ruth Bailey (she/her)

INTRODUCTION

The Nursing and Midwifery Council (NMC) code of practice (NMC 2018) clearly outlines the minimum standards that are required of every nurse and midwife on the professional register on a day-to-day basis, but what does 'being professional' really mean? Why is professionalism important? How do you become a professional? How do we recognise other professionals? What are the benefits and opportunities of being part of a professional community?

This chapter will aim to answer these questions by exploring some of the key components of professionalism and illustrating these with examples from practice.

It will highlight the facets of professional nursing and offer useful tips and practical resources to help you develop your own pathway towards professionalism beyond the NMC code of conduct.

> 'Be persistent, insistent & consistent and when you get resistance, seek assistance'.
>
> Dr. Joan Myers, OBE, FQNI

WHAT DO WE MEAN BY PROFESSIONALISM?

Professionalism is a term used to describe the attributes and behaviours shown by a person that inspire confidence and trust and actively demonstrate the values of nursing.

> 'It is working in a way that demonstrates compassionate and inclusive leadership and upholds the values and guiding principles your profession'.
>
> **Jason Warriner, FRCN, Director of care qualiy and governance**

In the IPOS Veracity Index published in 2022, the public voted nursing as the most trusted profession. It is important that we continue to practise our professional values so that we can uphold public faith and confidence in us. This section explores some of the fundamental values of nursing and looks at what these values might look like when they are put into practice.

> 'Being professional means being brave, having courage to advocate for patients, families, colleagues, and the profession even when others are silent. It's about doing the right thing, as well as doing things right!'
>
> **Evelyn Prodger, RN, QN, clinical services director**

Building professionalism doesn't happen overnight; it's a career-long journey that evolves over time and constantly develops with experience and reflection, and it can be a fantastic adventure! There are some tools that can be actively used to develop professionalism, and some of these are suggested in this chapter.

9 | NOTES ON PROFESSIONAL NURSING: BEYOND THE CODE

> What does professionalism look like? Picture the most professional nurse that you have worked with so far. What is it about them that made you select them for this exercise? What is it about them that you admire? What nursing values do they demonstrate? What have you learned from them? Do you think that you might be selected as someone else's example of a 'professional nurse'?
>
> _____
> _____
> _____
> _____
> _____

NURSING VALUES

'Compassion is not a passive emotion; it's an active force that drives us to make a difference'.—Mary Seacole

The Royal College of Nursing (RCN) updated its definition of nursing in September 2023 and said, 'Compassionate leadership is central to the provision and co-ordination of care informed by its values, integrity, and professional knowledge' (RCN 2023). This means that we need to be clear on what our shared nursing values are so that we can actively practise and develop them.

A decade ago, NHS England identified six core values for nursing, midwifery and care staff, known as the 6Cs (Department of Health 2012). These are care, compassion, competence, communication, courage and commitment. These values are the essence of nursing practice and outline the behaviours that the public can expect.

More recently, the chief nursing officer for England announced a new vision for nurses, midwives and nursing associates that identified five focus areas and two enablers, now known as 'The 7 Ps (Devereux 2023). The purpose of the vision was to give clear direction as to how the profession could work collaboratively to protect and promote the health of the nation in the current socioeconomic climate, both now and for the future.

Table 9.1 summarises the 7 Ps and gives examples of how this can be demonstrated in practice.

TABLE 9.1 THE 7 PS

7 Ps	What does it mean?	Examples in practice
Focus area 1 Protecting our planet	Nurses and midwives championing sustainability, advocating for those most affected by climate change Delivering lower-carbon care	Cycling to work/car-sharing initiatives Reducing unnecessary use of plastic gloves Switching patients from multidose inhalers to more environmentally friendly dry powder inhalers
Focus area 2 Prevention, protection promotion and reducing health inequalities	Maximising contribution across the life course, with focus on prevention, protection and wider determinants of health.	Supporting patients to increase movement and activity. Encouraging engagement and uptake of immunisation programmes. Initiatives that increase uptake of cervical screening for people with disabilities.
Focus area 3 Person-centred care	Person-centred care to be at the heart of practice, encouraging people to manage their health and care.	Nurse-led rough sleepers initiatives that work to encourage participation in health and social care. Multiprofessional programmes that support people with dementia to live rich and full lives.

TABLE 9.1 THE 7 PS—cont'd

7 Ps	What does it mean?	Examples in practice
Focus area 4 Public and patient safety	Recognising nursing and midwifery as a safety-critical profession, focused on quality safety, creating a culture where concerns are raised and acted upon.	Supportive serious adverse event reviews. Use of nurse metrics to review and act upon patient outcomes Working collaboratively with patient participant groups.
Focus area 5 Professional leadership and integration	Nurses and midwives using unique skills across the life course to drive better integration to meet the needs of patients and communities	Specialist midwives working with multiprofessional colleagues to support survivors of female genital mutilation. End-of-life care initiatives working with multiprofessional specialists and primary care to enable high-quality end-of-life care.
Enabler 1 People and workforce development	Nurses and midwives will have rewarding careers with access to lifelong learning. Health and well-being of the workforce to be prioritised.	Support and time for critical reflection Access to learning and development Support for mental health and suicide prevention.
Enabler 2 Professional culture	Promoting a culture of inclusivity which values evidence practice, research, digital data and technology.	Active promotion of equality, diversity and inclusion strategies. Provision of antiracist programmes Expanding research careers Expanding skills development in digital nursing

maintain physical, mental and spiritual health. It includes the building blocks of health such as eating a nutritious and balanced diet, staying hydrated, daily movement and exercise, engaging in national immunisation and screening programmes, maintaining dental health, accessing contraception, practising meditation, mindfulness or prayer, and engaging in faith-based or spiritual activities aligned with your personal values.

It also means building in time for rest and recuperation. The RCN's 'Rest, rehydrate, refuel' guidance published in 2018 reminds us of the importance of taking regular breaks and staying hydrated and well fuelled so that we can care effectively. Taking time to invest in health will ensure that you have enough energy to care for others and develop professionally; you will also be setting a great example!

There has been growing recognition that the emotional labour of nursing can take its toll on mental health, and the incidence of stress, anxiety, depression and serious mental illness has skyrocketed in during and after the COVID-19 pandemic. In 2021, the levels of sickness and absence due to stress and anxiety were 50% higher than in 2020 (NHS England 2023), and so, the need to take positive action on maintaining mental health has never been so crucial. Prevention is key, and investing time to promote good mental health is invaluable.

Mind is a national organisation that campaigns for support, understanding and respect for everyone who experiences a mental health problem. Its website is full of valuable resources to prevent poor mental health and to support those who experience it. It offers some practical tips, presented in the following box, which have shown to be effective in promoting mental well-being.

> **TIPS**
>
> Practical tips for mental well-being adapted from online resources at Mind.org:
>
> Connect: Connecting with others can help us feel valued and give a sense of community:
>
> - Ask a neighbour about their weekend.
> - Join a choir/book group/football team

TIPS—cont'd

Get active: Physical activity releases endorphins and can help us feel more positive:

- Have a brisk walk around the block.
- Join an exercise class/sports club.
- Cycle to work.
- Go for a swim.
- Put some music on and dance.

Take notice: Being mindful or savouring the moment can help identify moments of joy or gratitude and give your mind a rest:

- Take a moment to notice nature.
- Notice the different senses, sights, sounds and smells on the way to work.
- Notice how your body feels.
- List three things that you are currently grateful for.

Learn: Learning new skills can boost self-esteem and give a sense of investing in yourself:

- Sign up for a class.
- Have fun doing a puzzle.
- Learn a language.
- Read a chapter of a new book.
- Revisit a childhood passion.

Give: Giving back or doing something for others can boost feelings of self-worth:

- Offer a lift.
- Donate to a food bank.
- Fundraise for a charity.
- Host a tea party.
- Take part in a community clean-up.

The team at Shinymind has developed an award-winning evidence-based app designed specifically to support nurses in maintaining good mental health and well-being. Its interactive resources and toolkits have been shown to reduce stress and anxiety and build workplace resilience.

It is important that you take positive steps to ask for help from a healthcare professional if you notice a decline in mental health in yourself or others. Doing so means that you can access the expertise needed, and it will also help break down the stigma that surrounds mental illness.

> Are you getting regular breaks at work? Are you able to stay fuelled and hydrated at work? What are you doing for yourself, just for fun? What changes could you make to enhance your wellness?
>
> _____
>
> _____
>
> _____
>
> _____

MANAGING YOUR BOUNDARIES

The NMC code of practice (NMC 2018) requires us all to work within our scope of professional practice, and this means, unless we are training and under direct supervision, we only undertake procedures for which we are confident that we have achieved the required competence to carry it out safely. Working within our scope of practice means keeping both our patients and us safe.

THE NMC SAYS

13 Recognise and work within the limits of your competence.

It's important to know what your boundaries of practice are and be able to say no, negotiate or ask for help if asked to do something outside your current scope of practice.

Developing skills in assertiveness can be helpful. Assertiveness is defined as 'promoting my rights, while respecting the rights of others' (Dickson 2022). It is the skill of stating your position or asking for what you need, in a style that is clear and balanced, while being respectful of the feelings of the person you are talking to.

> **CASE STUDY**
>
> Elliott is a newly qualified nurse in general practice, has recently attended a course in ear irrigation and has undertaken the skill once under supervision. The practice manager informs him that his colleague is off sick and has a clinic full of patients who need ear irrigation; they all have waited several weeks for the appointment and are desperate for the procedure. Elliott is keen to step up and contribute to the service pressures. He doesn't want to let the patients down, but he doesn't feel he is competent to carry out the procedure alone, as he knows it carries a risk of infection and perforation.
>
> He politely tells the practice manager that he is not yet confident to carry out the procedure unsupervised and asks that the appointments are rebooked to ensure the procedure is carried out safely.

In the context of increasing workload pressures and short staffing, you may find yourself under pressure to stay late working over your contracted hours or do extra shifts on the bank to help. It is important that you only do so if it is convenient to you, it brings you personal benefit and it is fully paid!

It can be very difficult to say no, but you may need to do so to protect your boundaries and your personal energy and resources. Saying no with kindness is a useful life skill and takes some practice.

> **TIPS**
>
> Practical tips on assertive communication:
>
> Recognise the other person's difficulty: 'I realise this is a tricky situation and must make it very difficult for you'.
>
> State your case: 'I'm sorry that I am unable to stay late tonight, as I have another commitment'.
>
> State what you can reasonably offer (if you can): 'I could ask my colleague who does bank shifts and may be available/I could perhaps change my shift next week/I am sorry; I don't have extra capacity right now'.
>
> Close the communication: 'I do hope you manage to find someone and that the situation isn't too stressful'.

CHALLENGING POOR PRACTICE

> *'Sometimes being professional means not going with the flow, recognising something isn't right and being vocal'.*
>
> **Wendie Smith, QN**

Despite widespread commitment to high standards of care, poor practice can occur in any setting where care is being delivered. Poor practice can be defined as treatment or care that falls below expected standards or is delivered outside national guidance.

> **THE NMC SAYS**
>
> 16 Act without delay if you believe that there is a risk to patient safety or public protection.

Examples of poor practice include staff forgetting to introduce themselves, leaving confidential information in view, failing to maintain privacy when washing patients, not fully explaining procedures, breaches in patient confidentiality and not giving opportunities for patients to be involved in their own care.

No healthcare professional deliberately intends to deliver poor care, and there are complex reasons why this happens. It may be that workload pressures result in taking shortcuts, or it may be that lack of education means staff are simply not aware of best practice or that the poor practice has just become the cultural norm. Whatever the root cause, poor practice is likely to continue unless it is challenged.

Part of being professional is building the strength and courage to act when standards are not maintained, but this can feel awkward and challenging, and using a framework to structure the conversation can help.

One helpful framework is the use of the mnemonic RISC, which stands for report, impact, specify and close. The following box demonstrates how the RISC framework can be used to structure a conversation to challenge practice.

> **R Report the activity**
>
> *'I couldn't help noticing that when you left your clinic room, the door was open, and the computer screen was unlocked. I know that you are busy, and it is easy to forget...'*
>
> **I Explain the impact**
>
> *'but this worried me because that patient's notes were on display, anyone could have read them and that would be a breach of her confidentiality'.*
>
> **S Specify what needs to happen**
>
> *'Please could I ask you to lock your screen or your clinic door so that the notes are kept private?'*
>
> **C Close the conversation**
>
> *'Thank you for taking that on board'.*

There may be times when you may not feel resilient enough to have a difficult conversation or you simply feel out of your depth. It is important to acknowledge this and seek help. If you don't feel that you can approach your supervisor or a senior nurse, you may want to contact the local freedom to speak guardian who you can approach in confidence.

> Think of an example of poor practice that you have witnessed but did not challenge.
>
> Some suggestions include:
>
> - A colleague who did not wash their hands
> - A colleague making an inappropriate joke
> - A team member coming back late from a break
> - A colleague who did not follow a procedure properly
>
> Now go back through the RISC framework and use it to give the feedback that you would have liked to give at the time of the incident. What will you **Report**? How will you explain the **Impact**, what change would you like to **Specify** and how would you like to **Close** the conversation?
>
> _____
> _____
> _____
> _____
> _____

Responding to Criticism from Others

There will be times when your practice will be challenged, and this can feel very awkward and uncomfortable, but it can be extremely valuable in developing your professional practice. It is worth remembering that none of us are likely to develop our skills if our only feedback is glowing praise! Learning to handle criticism is a very useful skill and can be used to enhance our personal practice.

> **TIPS**
>
> Tips for handling criticism:
>
> - View the criticism as a gift and thank the person who gives it to you.
> - The feedback may be painful or unfair, but through it, you have gained an insight into how the giver of it views your practice, and this has value.
> - Keep the feedback in context.
> - The feedback is the observation of one person. Remember that the feedback is just that; it is not a comment on your character or your whole career.
> - Decide what you do with the feedback.
> - Think about the feedback that you have been given, and decide if it is valid or not. If you are uncertain of its validity, it may be useful to discuss with a trusted mentor. Sharing with a friend will make you feel better, but it may not help your learning.
> - If the feedback is valid, you may be able to use it to improve your practice or modify your behaviour in some way.
> - If the feedback is unfair, then use it to open a discussion on your differences in opinion.
> - You may decide to mull the feedback over and give it more thought, or you may decide to disregard it. It is your feedback and taking ownership and deciding what to do will give you control.

LEARNING FROM MISTAKES

'Mistakes are the portal of discovery'

—James Joyce

The RCN defines nursing as a 'safety-critical' profession (RCN 2023), and this term is used to describe a system where failure or malfunction can result in serious injury or death. Nursing expertise is critical in ensuring safety, preventing errors and contributing to positive patient outcomes.

Routine activities such as checking the temperature of the drug fridge, completing hand-washing audits and monitoring the rate of patient slips, trips and falls are all examples of nursing activities that contribute to reducing risk and maintaining safety on a day-to-day basis.

Nobody wants to make a mistake, particularly if it results in harm to a patient or colleague, but making mistakes is inevitable, and learning to respond to a mistake and manage the fallout is an important professional skill.

The depth and breadth of nursing practice are wide and represent enormous scope for making mistakes, and their seriousness will be assessed based on risk of potential or actual harm. According to an NMC report (NMC 2024), the mistakes that most are most seen in fitness to practice proceedings are those related to patient care (23%), prescribing and medicines management (16%) and recordkeeping (13%).

Learning from mistakes can inform our future practice and enable us to change our procedures to reduce the likelihood of them happening again. This can be a powerful development tool, but it can also be a painful process, and it can be useful to have a strategy ready to use to help you manage the situation. It can also be helpful to talk it through with a trusted mentor to support you in managing any emotional distress.

> **TIPS**
>
> Tips for managing mistakes:
>
> **Report the mistake.**
> First, acknowledge the mistake, and report it to the senior nurse on duty as soon as you can. This will help you shoulder the responsibility for putting things right, and it will also help you manage the emotional burden of making a mistake.
>
> **Own the mistake and apologise.**
> Owning the mistake and apologising without apportioning blame can be extremely powerful.
>
> 'I am really sorry, but I made a drug error and have given 1 g of IV amoxicillin instead of 500 mg' demonstrates much greater

> **TIPS—cont'd**
>
> professionalism than 'I've only had a bank nurse with me, I've been so stressed, and now I realise I've made a drug error; I told you staffing wasn't safe.'
>
> **Take action to address the mistake.**
> We have a responsibility to open and honest and tell our patients what has gone wrong under 'duty of candour'. It can be difficult to tell a patient that we have made a mistake, but they usually really appreciate the honesty and courage shown, and it can be very powerful in restoring trust. 'Tom, I am so sorry, I have given you double the dose of the antibiotic prescribed by mistake; I want to carry out some observations to make sure you are okay'.
>
> **Document the mistake**
> Record the facts of the mistake using your organisation's reporting system. This is known as Datix or serious adverse event. It is helpful to record the facts of what happened when, and record what action was taken at the time. This will assist any investigation that may be necessary and can help pinpoint what went wrong so that mechanisms can be put in place to avoid it happening again.
>
> **Write a brief reflection**
> It can be hard not to dwell on a mistake, and it is easy to ruminate, replaying events in your head. Writing a reflection is a really good way of making sense of the incident so that you can take the learning from it and move on. It can be helpful to think about what went wrong, what went well and what practical steps you might take personally to avoid repetition. Demonstrating insight is a powerful way of communicating the learning from the event and using it to deepen your professional understanding.
>
> **Congratulate yourself**
> Remind yourself that making mistakes is part of being human and part of professional growth. Recognise that the mistake has been managed, and give yourself permission to move on and congratulate yourself for making sense of what has happened.

> 'While I was working in a sexual health clinic, I saw a patient who asked for Levonelle 1500 mcg for emergency contraception. I issued this under a patient group direction (PGD), and as I was inputting details of the medication in the electronic patent record, I realised to my horror that the Levonelle had expired a month ago and would not be effective. I told the matron what I had done, and she helped me put it right. As a prescriber, she wrote a patient specific direction (PSD) for a second dose of the medication and reassured me this was safe.
>
> I called the patient back, explained what had happened and issued another dose.
>
> I completed a Datix form and shared it at our team meeting.
>
> Obviously, I should have checked the expiry date before giving the drug, and the clinic should not have had expired drugs on the shelves. A healthcare assistant suggested a new system of checking the dates of drugs on the first of every month to reduce the risk of it happening again.
>
> I was really helped knowing that a change of practice had come out of my mistake, reducing the risk for everyone, and I wrote the whole incident up as a reflection for my NMC portfolio'.
>
> *Ruth Bailey, ANP, sexual health*

DEVELOPING AS AN ADVOCATE

Acting as a patient advocate is a fundamental part of nursing. Nsiah et al. (2019) describe advocacy as being the patient's voice and acting on their behalf to ensure their needs are met. This can mean supporting patients to voice their opinions and concerns and stepping in to act on their behalf if they are unable to.

THE NMC SAYS

3.4 Act as an advocate for the vulnerable, challenging poor practice and discriminatory attitudes and behaviour relating to their care.

Being an advocate means being their champion, fighting their corner and standing up for their rights. If you have been on a clinical placement, you will have almost certainly acted as an advocate for a patient in your care.

> **CASE STUDY**
>
> The following are a few examples of how nurses can advocate for patients.
>
> Ashanti asks a physio if she can visit later in the day when her patients' painkillers have had a chance to work.
>
> Taj asks a doctor on a ward round to wait for him to put his patients' hearing aids in before starting her discussion.
>
> Mae asks if her patient's medication can be changed to a liquid form, as the tablets are too big to swallow and are sticking in her throat.
>
> Robin asks the ward manager for permission for her patient's daughter to stay beyond visiting time, as she has travelled a long distance.

Nurses may also advocate for groups of patients, for societal change and for nursing practice. Nursing can be an effective force of social justice, and by working collaboratively, we can use our skills in advocacy and our clinical expertise and professional credibility to highlight unmet needs or gaps in care to raise awareness and campaign for change. Connecting as a profession enables us to raise awareness, champion a cause, exert political pressure to shape policy and effect change.

There are many examples of how nurses have successfully advocated for groups of patients and for groups of nurses demonstrating the value that we bring.

The following box contains examples of nurse advocacy for patients:

#Cervical screening awareness Jo's Trust	Jo's Trust was established to raise awareness and provide resources and support for those affected by cervical cancer. Every year in June, it works with nurses to promote screening, raising awareness and encouraging activities such as drop-in clinics and open days.
Dame Elizabeth Aionwu advocating for patients with sickle cell	Dame Elizabth Aionwu became the first sickle cell nurse specialist in the United Kingdom and helped establish the Sickle Cell Society, the only UK society to support those with sickle cell disorder and to improve quality of life.

The following box shows examples of nurse's advocating for nursing:

Queen's Nursing Institute	Advocates for community nurses, campaigns to ensure that high-quality community nursing is available where and when it is needed. Highlights the essential roles that community nursing plays, sets standards of practice, offers a wide range of development programmes. Offers practical support.
Mental Health Nurses Day Feb 21st	Introduced by RCN Mental Health Forum 2019 to respond to a drop in numbers of mental health nurses. The campaign celebrates the contribution of mental health nurses, showcases their work, debunks myths and encourages interest in the speciality.

Participating in professional advocacy can begin with very simple steps. It may be signing up to a mailing list for a cause close to your heart. It can be signing a petition calling for change; it can be a matter of writing a letter to an MP or participating in a digital awareness campaign. There are many opportunities to complete online surveys that will ask for your experience or opinion, and this is an effective way of voicing your experience to influence change. For example, in 2022, results from the *Nursing Times* survey for newly qualified nurses demonstrated a lack of support at the start of their careers and campaigned for greater preceptorship and support (Mitchell 2022).

Connecting with other nurses in your chosen speciality or who share your experience or interests is a great way of keeping up to date, sharing ideas or innovations, problem solving and supporting each other. Your own organisation may facilitate specialists' forums or journal clubs as an employee benefit.

The RCN offers a range of professional nursing forums that are free for members to join. The forums promote best practice, publish evidence-based guidance and provide a professional network free to members.

> **When did you last act as an advocate for a patient? When did you last advocate for nursing? What one step would you like to take towards developing advocacy?**
>
> _____
>
> _____
>
> _____
>
> _____

EQUALITY DIVERSITY AND INCLUSION: DEVELOPING ALLYSHIP

'Anyone has the potential to be an ally. Allies recognise that although they're not a member of an underinvested or oppressed communities they support, they make a concerted effort to understand the struggle, every day'.

—Roxane Gray

Under the Equality Act 2010, it is against the law to discriminate against anyone on the grounds of age, disability, gender reassignment, marriage and civil partnership pregnancy and maternity, race, religion, belief, sex or sexual orientation. However, members of these groups do experience discrimination, and a key nursing principle is to champion inclusivity and inclusion (RCN 2023) both for our patients and our colleagues. Our workforce is enriched by our diversity, and there is evidence to show that fair treatment of staff results in safer care for patients (King's Fund 2020).

In a profession that values kindness, compassion, individuality and justice, we have a responsibility to act as allies, defined as someone who champions an underrepresented or marginalised group while not being a member of that group themselves. Principles of allyship extend to all underrepresented groups valuing and supporting people to be their authentic selves.

Lesbian Gay Bisexual Transgender Queer (Questioning)+

According to Stonewall (2018), over a Third LGBTQ+ people still feel that they must hide who they are at work, and one in eight would not feel confident to report homophobic or biphobic bullying. We know that nurses need to feel psychologically safe to deliver the best care, and so, it's important to support our LGBTQ+ colleagues to flourish. Avoiding making assumptions, using the right pronoun and using the gender-neutral term 'partner' are ways to recognise diversity (Gilmore 2023). Recognising LGBTQ+ champions and role models and celebrating pride in nursing are visible ways we can support, affirm and value colleagues from the LGBTQ+ community.

Tackling Racism

Despite having one of the most diverse workforces in the public sector, we know that racism exists in healthcare (Kings Fund 2020). Data from the workforce race equality standard (NHS WRES 2022) have demonstrated staff from the global majority are less likely to be promoted than their White colleagues and reported that one in four have experienced harassment and bullying in the workplace.

As registered professionals, we all have a responsibility to challenge discrimination and work with our employers towards zero tolerance. In 2022 the NHS Confederation developed a practical resource toolkit for combatting racism based on a framework of authentic inclusion, challenging racism, challenging leadership, and caring and belonging. This offers a range of resources to deepen our understanding and equip us for challenge.

As humans, we all have our own biases and prejudices, and the first step in authentic allyship is recognising this, taking responsibility and working to unlearn behaviours which perpetuate the situation. This means listening to the accounts of people who have experienced racism, believing it and opening our eyes to injustice (Trueland 2020).

There are many reasons why white nurses may find it difficult to discuss race or culture. They may deny or minimise the issue, they may fail to take responsibility for it or they may be worried about causing upset or saying the wrong thing. Listening to colleagues and creating a safe space, being curious, asking about experiences, calling out microaggressions and being willing to challenge discrimination can be positive steps towards allyship.

The following box shows the 'A's of Authentic Allyship', presented by Yvonne Coghill in The Pemberton Lecture 2020, and now used in many antiracist toolkits (Trueland 2020).

Appreciate

Fully appreciate the benefits of diversity and genuinely and demonstrably work towards making the workplace more equitable.

> **Appetite**
>
> Do you have the appetite to immerse yourself in the complex emotive world of race equality?

Continued

> **Ask**
>
> Ask questions about race, be curious, read. Learn and educate yourself.
>
> **Accept**
>
> Accept there is a problem—more data isn't needed.
>
> **Acknowledge**
>
> Openly acknowledge that the problem needs to be dealt with.
>
> **Apologise**
>
> Express sympathy that racism is affecting people of certain races.
>
> **Assume**
>
> Don't! Instead develop informed views by seeking to understand individuals.
>
> **Action**
>
> Take demonstrable steps to establish equality and be accountable.

EMBRACING NEURODIVERSITY

Neurodiversity is an umbrella term given to encompass a range of naturally occurring neurological conditions that each characterise differences in learning styles, challenges and skills. The most common of these include dyslexia, dyspraxia, autism spectrum disorders and attention deficit hyperactivity disorder. An estimated 10%–15% of the population is thought to be neurodiverse (RCN 2022); there are thought to be more neurodiverse people in healthcare, and I am one of them!

Nurses with neurodiverse conditions will have challenges, but we also have valuable skills, insights and talents that neuronormative nurses don't have. Simple adjustments can result in huge differences for neurodiverse nurses, and supporting us to perform at our best may result in better care for patients.

The following box shows examples of reasonable adjustments:

- Asking a colleague what support they need to learn a new skill
- Use of dictation software
- Providing large print
- Preventing sensory overload
- Giving extra time for procedures
- Giving a predictable shift pattern
- Providing altered lighting

LIFELONG LEARNING

Part of developing professionalism is active commitment to lifelong learning to develop our knowledge and skills. The context of healthcare is always changing, our evidence base is constantly being developed, the guidance on which we base our practice will evolve and so, the need for education is lifelong. Engaging as an active participant in ongoing learning is a good habit to develop; it brings rich rewards, and it can be great fun!

It is worth thinking about the options you have available to access ongoing learning so that you can set up your own system and embed learning habits that will serve you throughout your career.

PRACTICAL REFLECTION

Reflecting on practice and making sense of an experience is the foundation of professional growth. The NMC states that reflection is a way to make sense of a situation and how it affects us; it helps identify areas for further development, fosters learning from other professionals and enables us to consider how to put changes or improvement into action (NMC 2019). All registered nurses are required to submit five reflective accounts as a requirement for revalidation, and the NMC provides a template to structure this; it can be useful to get in the habit of writing them as you go along. It helps develop reflective skills, and it means you are ahead of the game when revalidation comes around.

There is compelling evidence that access to supervision is linked to enhanced quality of care, patient safety and staff well-being, and there may be opportunities through your employers or networks to engage in reflective practice in action learning sets, clinical supervision or within multiprofessional teams. Working with others can give you a wide breadth of insight as you learn from the experience of others. There are increasing opportunities to access supervision online, widening access to this effective learning tool.

KEEPING UP TO DATE WITH THE NURSING LITERATURE

Many healthcare trusts will have their own library that will operate a knowledge share alert that is a free service for employees. As an employee, you join the library and list your interests, and the library staff will send you a monthly round-up of a list of publications that match your interests, updating you, with minimal effort on your part.

Members of the RCN will have access to the UK's largest collection of nursing literature and can access nursing journals free of charge. The RCN library staff will also undertake literature searches for registered nurses free of charge. You may wish to sign up for BrowZine, a platform that allows you to access e-journals on your device.

> **THE NMC SAYS**
>
> **22.3** Keep your knowledge and skills up to date, taking part in appropriate and regular learning and professional development activities that aim to maintain and develop your competence and improve your performance.

USING SOCIAL MEDIA

The use of social media offers a wealth of opportunities to connect with nurses who share your interests by enabling you to become connected and join a community of nurses with a shared passion. Joining a Facebook/X group, Instagram account or email list will give you instant access to expertise in your field and will alert you to updated guidance, practical resources and forthcoming learning opportunities. Since the COVID-19 pandemic, there has been a huge increase in the provision of online webinars, many of which are free.

ACCESSING LEARNING EVENTS

Undertaking courses of specific study or attending conferences is extremely valuable in enriching your nursing knowledge and providing networking opportunities. If you can attend a learning event, you might want to consider how you will share your experiences and learning with colleagues, either formally or informally. Attending events can be costly, so it is worth exploring the many funding opportunities that are available. Each will have their own specific application criteria, and it's worth investigating these.

The following box shows organisations that offer grants and scholarships for nurses:

The Burdett Trust	The trust was established in 2002 with the aim of providing charitable grants to support nurse-led projects to make significant improvements in patient care. A wide range of grants aim to support positive outcomes in such areas as research, leadership, health advocacy, diversity inclusivity and well-being.
The Cavell Trust	The charity supports nurses, midwives and healthcare assistants, working or retired, in times of personal or financial hardship, providing emotional support, practical advice and financial relief in the form of one-off grants or emergency funding.
The Florence Nightingale Foundation	The foundation aims to support nurses and midwives to improve care and save lives through building leadership capacity and capability. It provides a wide range of prestigious leadership scholarships, development programmes and online learning opportunities.

Continued

FSRH	The Faculty is a multi-disciplinary professional organisation providing clinical guidance, education and leadership in SRH. It provides a number of bursaries for its annual conferences and a membership fund that can be accessed by members to fund educational programmes in SRH.
The QNI	The QNI is dedicated to improving the nursing care of people in their own homes and communities. It provides a telephone helpline and financial help for community services. It offers a wide range of leadership and development programmes for community nurses and a bursary for those undertaking the QNI aspiring leader's programme.
The Royal College of Nursing Foundation	The foundation aims to strengthen nursing, midwifery and social care to support the health and well-being of the public. It provides hardship grants and a wide range of grants to support education, research and practice development. You don't need to be an RCN member to apply!

FSRH, The Faculty of Sexual and Reproductive Health; *QNI,* Queen's Nurse Institute; *SRH,* sexual and reproductive health.

MAKING MENTORSHIP WORK FOR YOU

'A good mentor teaches with approachability and willingness to learn themselves. They develop professional relationships and utilise resources to ensure their student has a good learning experience'.

Verity Scourfield, RN, NQN

'The good mentor has been the one that saw the vision passion and drive I have, and who helped me direct it in the right way, rather than hinder my growth mindset. It's difficult

finding such mentors but I've been lucky to meet a few who have supported me through my formative years in nursing'.

Cyzel Gomes, RN, NQN

Mentors are not just for student nurses; they are there to help coach support and navigate throughout your professional career. Working with a skilled mentor who you trust can transform and enrich your practice. Mentoring doesn't need to be a formal process; it may be a nurse you admire and identify as a role model whose opinion and advice you seek on an ad hoc basis. Good mentors can offer you constructive feedback, guide you and create opportunities for your future development.

You may choose to act as a mentor yourself or for other students or colleagues. Acting as a mentor can challenge you to sharpen your own nursing knowledge and provide experience in teaching, coaching and offering constructive feedback, all of which will enhance your own practice.

CONNECTING WITH A GLOBAL COMMUNITY

'The real value of being part of a global community is to enable nurses to show their collective impact, demonstrating leadership and our unique contribution to health and social care that makes a difference to the lives of people, communities and countries'.

Jason Warriner, FRCN, Director of care quality and governance Cranstoun

Nursing is a career that presents infinite opportunities. As nurses, we are members of a global community recognisable by our shared professional values and united through our commitment to care. Our nursing education provides us with a foundation of transferable skills that gives us a passport to move across specialities, organisations and geographical borders.

Part of developing professionalism is about connecting with our colleagues across the world so that we can pool our collective knowledge, share our learning and work collaboratively to expand our ability to protect and promote nursing and ultimately work to improve global health.

The International Council of Nurses (ICN) is a federation of more than 130 nursing associations across the world that represents over 28 million nurses. Working together with member organisations, it provides a framework for nurses to work together on shared concerns such as ethical recruitment, improving nurse retention and strengthening nurse leadership.

> **CASE STUDY**
>
> **Nursing Now Challenge**
>
> The Nursing Now Challenge 2021 was a global nursing project launched by the Burdett Trust in collaboration with the World Health Organization and the ICN. It was set up to raise the profile and status of nursing by empowering student and early-career nurses to act as practitioners, advocates and leaders to address the health issues in their communities. It created a dynamic global network, providing opportunities in leadership development and shared learning and peer support for nurses. The Nursing Now Challenge has recently joined with the global health network to launch The 1000 Challenge: Research, Leadership, Impact, to support and equip nurse's to address health inequalities across the world.

Working in global partnership has enabled nurses to come together to tackle some of the major health challenges that we currently face, such as addressing the health consequences of climate change through greener practices, influencing the uptake of immunisation and addressing the aftermath of COVID-19 in communities across the world. Through our collective professional activism, we have the opportunity to strengthen nursing and enhance our ability to impact health and well-being across the world.

> **TIPS**
>
> Tips for engaging in global nursing:
>
> - Sign up for the ICN newsletter.
> - Follow a global nurse leader on social media.
> - Complete an ICN e-learning module at ICN-eLearning.
> - Explore your university's international connections.
> - Connect with an international colleague.
> - Join in the celebrations on International Nurses Day, May 12.

CONCLUSION

Becoming a registered nurse means that we join a professional community with shared core values and standards of conduct. This brings responsibilities but also endless possibilities for self-development, discovery and reward. This chapter has outlined those core values and discussed how we might practice them.

It has encouraged nurses to look after their own health and well-being to be able to care for others, and it has discussed some of the challenges faced in developing professional practice beyond the code.

Space for reader's own reflection:
___
___
___
___
___
___

REFERENCES

Coghill, Y., 2020. Pemberton Lecture 2020: A Review, The University of Sheffield.

Davies, R., 2020. Promoting and supporting healthy eating among nurses. Nurs. Stand. 35 (8), 45–50. doi:10.7748/ns.2020.e11535

Department of Health. 2012. Compassion in Practice. https://www.england.nhs.uk/wp-content/uploads/2012/12/compassion-in-practice.pdf

Devereux, E., 2023. New 7P's for nursing unveiled as part of CNO strategy. Nursing Times Published online https://nursingtimes.net/leadership/new-7ps-for-nursing-unveiledas-part-of-cno-strategy-16-11-2023/

Staff: Our Vision and Strategy. https://www.england.nhs.uk/wp-content/uploads/2012/12/compassion-in-practice.pdf

Dickson, A., 2022. A Woman in Your Own Right: The Art of Assertive, Clear and Honest Communication, Duckworth Books.

Gilmore, J.P., Dainton, M., Halpin, N., 2024. Authentic allyship for gender minorities. J. Nurs. Scholarsh. 56, 5–8.

Imperial College Health Care NHS Trust 2023 Being an Ally Toolkit. https://www.imperial.nhs.uk/-/media/website/about-us/how-we-work/equality-and—diversity/allyship-toolkit_14_03.pdf

King's Fund. 2020. The Courage of Compassion; Supporting Nurses and Midwives to Deliver High Quality Care. The King's Fund. kingsfund.org.uk [Accessed September 2023]

King's Fund. 2020. Workforce race inequalities and inclusion in NHS Providers. The King's Fund. kingsfund.org.uk [Accessed September 2023]

Mitchell, G., 2022. Campaign Calls for all NRN to receive 'vital' preceptorship. Nurs. Times 118 (2), 6–7.

Nurse and Midwifery Council. 2018. The Code: Professional Standards of Practice and Behaviour for Nurses, Midwives and Nursing Associates. https://www.nmc.org.uk/standards/code/

NHS England. 2023. Working Together to Prevent Suicide in the NHS Workforce: A National Suicide Prevention Tool Kit for England. https://www.england.nhs.uk/long-read/working-together-to-prevent-suicide-in-the-nhs-workforce/

NHS England. 2022. Workforce Race and Equality Standard. https://www.england.nhs.uk/publication/nhs-workforce-race-equality-standard-2022/ [Accessed September 2023]

NMC. 2024. Annual Fitness to practice Report. https://nmc.org.uk/globalassets/sitedocuments/annual_reports_and_accounts/ftpannualreports/2024-ftp-/annual-fitness-to-practice-report-2023-2024.pdf

Nsiah, C., Siakwa, M., Ninnoni, J.P.K., 2019. Registered Nurses descriptions of patient advocacy in the clinical setting. Nurs. Open. 6 (3), 1124–1132. doi:10.1002/nop2.307

Ross, A., Yang, L., Wehrlen, L., et al., 2019. Nurses and health-promoting self-care: do we practice what we preach? J. Nurs. Manag. 27 (3), 599–608. doi:10.1111/jonm.12718

Royal College of Nursing. 2023. Definition and Principles of Nursing. Royal College of Nursing. rcn.org.uk. [Accessed September 2023]

Royal College of Nursing. 2022. Neurodiversity Pocket Guide. What is neurodiversity? | Neurodiversity RCN | Peer Support Service | Royal College of Nursing.

RCN. 2024. Celebrating Mental Health Nurses Day. https://www.rcn.org.uk/news-and-events/Blogs/celebrating-mental-health-nurses-day-210224 [Accessed November 2024]

Royal College on Nursing. 2018. Rest, Rehydrate and Refuel Campaign. https://www.rcn.org.uk/magazines/Activists/2018/March/Rest-rehydrate-refuel. [Accessed September 2023]

Stonewall. 2018. LGBT in Britain-Work Report. https:// www.stonewall.org.uk/resources/lgbt-britain-work-report-2018

Trueland, J., 2020. How you can tackle causal racism and microaggression in the NHS. Nurs. Stand. https://rcni.com/nursing-standard/features/

World Health Organization. 2021. Self Care Interventions for Health. WHO, Geneva Switzerland.